BASIC PRINCIPLES OF TOTAL HEALTH

Harmonious Integration of Body, Mind, and Spirit
2024 Edition

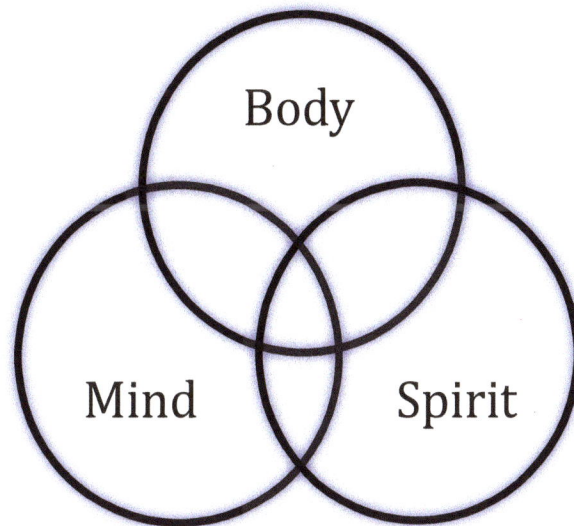

Body

Mind   Spirit

featuring

The Hierarchy of Nutrients

Jim Sharps, N.D., H.D., Dr. NSc.

Copyright © 2024 Jim Sharps, N.D., H.D., Dr. NSc
Copyright © 2024 TEACH Services, Inc.
ISBN-13: 978-1-4796-1694-7 (Paperback)
ISBN-13: 978-1-4796-1787-6 (Spiral)
ISBN-13: 978-1-4796-1695-4 (ePub)

For further information, contact:
International Institute of Original Medicine, P. O. Box 311, Smithfield, VA 23431
Or visit https://iiomonline.org/

Cover and Text Design: Diane Baier, D.Zyn Co.

Edited by Textworks and Drs. Jim and Elisa Sharps

First Printing: 1995
Millennium Edition: 2000
Third Printing: 2006
Fourth Printing: 2011
Fifth Printing: 2024

Printed by

TEACH Services, Inc.
PUBLISHING
www.TEACHServices.com • (800) 367-1844

Table of Contents

Table of Figures

List of Tables

Foreword

Medicine for the 21st century is going to place individuals at the core of its success and in the role of primary responsibility for their own health. In the highest form of health care, we place lifestyle first as both the cause of and correction for disease. Individually, we should look at the way we live as being the primary factor creating our health and vitality or lack of these positive attributes. Basic Preventive Medicine includes five important lifestyle keys:

1. Nutrition – eating a balanced and wholesome diet by focusing on natural foods, ideally eaten close to their harvest, i.e., seasonal nutrition.
2. Exercise – following a regular and varied program of stretching for flexibility, weight training for strength, and aerobic activity for endurance – all geared toward aiding relaxation and revitalization.
3. Sleep – getting the right number of hours of deep and restful sleep on a regular basis to recharge our body batteries and maintain immune strength and overall health.
4. Stress management – learning to relax and take life in stride, being able to deal with stresses at home and work and finding time to have fun at play, as well as being productive.
5. Attitude – maintaining a positive orientation toward life and its challenges is important to health and success. Attitude often underlies the desire to practice the first four lifestyle keys in giving yourself the best, because you want to love your body and care for it optimally.

In medical care and particularly in *health* care, an approach that is wise and that really works involves a treatment hierarchy of lifestyle first, natural therapies next, allopathic prescription medicine next, and other more invasive therapies as a last resort. However, in acute care medicine and for lifesaving heroics, Western medicine does not have an equal. Yet, most problems are not of that variety; they are vague aches and pains, fatigue, and a wide variety of chronic problems that come from decades of improper living.

Now, this is what the knowledgeable Dr. Jim Sharps is going to tell you about in the *Basic Principles of Total Health.* He is going to guide you through the many ways to follow these keys to preventing disease. He is going to inform you clearly and simply about the ideal diet; about the importance of exercise and rest; about air, water, and sunlight; and about an ancient, yet newly revitalized area of electromagnetic healing capabilities and how all of this can help you to improve your health and that of your family.

Dr. Sharps is going to provide you with a clear picture of how to create Total Health— Body, Mind, and Spirit. And I can assure you that if you listen to the good doctor, it can change your life and provide you with greater health.

I have read this book. It makes sense; it is not complicated. It is not authoritarian but gives you the support you need to make a difference. And I shall assure you, because I see it every day in my practice, that when you make changes in your lifestyle (even though this is not always easy), you are going to make a positive difference in your health, vitality, life, and longevity.

Good luck, but you won't need it if you follow the guidelines of natural living and take care of yourself.

Elson M. Haas, M.D.

Dr. Elson M. Hass is a physician who, over the last 25 years of practice, has developed the system of integrated health care. He is the founder and medical director of the Preventive Medical Center of Marin, an integrated healthcare facility in San Rafael, California. He is also the author of many books, including the highly acclaimed *Staying Healthy with Nutrition* and, his latest book, *The Detox Diet*.

About the Author

Dr. Jim Sharps is a Naturopathic Doctor, with additional doctorates in Herbal Medicine and Nutritional Science. He specializes in corrective nutrition, lifestyle evaluation, and natural health education. Dr. Sharps maintains a private practice in Columbia, Maryland where he conducts both onsite and telephone consultations. Also, he is President and Chief Executive Officer of the International Institute of Original Medicine, a distance learning school, that offers both certifications (Nutrition, Herbology, Medical Missionary, and Health Practitioner) and degree programs (Bachelor, Master's and Doctorate level curriculums in natural health). He lectures extensively on natural health to a broad spectrum of audiences including corporations, schools, and support groups.

His natural health focus began as a journey to understand and remedy several personal health challenges he experienced over thirty years ago, including allergies, respiratory problems, and chronic lower back problems. The New York native is no longer shackled by these earlier challenges and enjoys exceptionally good health, sporting with his two youngest pre-teen sons.

Dr. Sharps' studies, training, and education span a broad spectrum of disciplines, beyond Nutrition and Herbology, which include Acupressure, Shiatsu, Reflexology, Applied Kinesiology, Magnetic Therapy, Supervised Fasting, Yoga, Martial Arts, Self-Healing, Vision Training, Hydrotherapy, and several Therapeutic Massage techniques. He lectures extensively on natural health to a broad spectrum of audiences including corporations, schools, and support groups.

Dr. Sharps is the former President of the Board of Directors of the Self-Healing Research Foundation in San Francisco and a Director of the International Society of Naturopathy. He is the Founder and Executive Director of Integrated Health Therapies, a natural health services center in Oakland, California specializing in corrective nutrition, colon hydrotherapy, therapeutic massage, health education, and other health services. In addition, he holds an MBA in Marketing and Computer Methodology, as well as a BA in Economics. He worked for over twenty years in the information technology field for Fortune 500 and smaller companies. His extensive health training and knowledge combined with his corporate business background offer unique perspectives for business professionals. His contagious enthusiasm makes natural health both an enjoyable and informative experience.

Naturopathy: Purpose and Practice

Naturopathy is the oldest healing system in the world! It emphasizes the curative powers of nature. Naturopathic physicians work to restore and support the body's healing ability using various modalities, including nutrition, exercise, rest, herbal medicine, homeopathic medicine, oriental medicine, and therapeutic massage. The Naturopath is a Doctor of Natural Healing and an expert on optimum lifestyle issues.

Naturopathy is applied to suspend or slow down the aging process! Disease is understood in many instances as a natural method of eliminating waste and correcting other ailments within the body. The body usually responds remarkably well to natural treatment. The Naturopath is able to educate and recommend a course of action, which usually results in restoring a healthy, normal body and mind. Education, prevention, and a natural lifestyle are at the core of Natural Healing.

Nutrition is an important factor in natural healing! Many natural foods are healing agents. While many natural substances and herbs are used in natural healing, if the body is sick and full of accumulated waste, even the best foods available may not be indicated or effective until the poisons and waste have been removed. The result of eliminating waste from the body, or detoxifying, and then nourishing the body is the improved foundation of metabolic processes required for optimum health. Practicing naturopathy encourages and promotes personal responsibility, self-care, self-motivation, education, and a more disciplined lifestyle.

The three basic principles of Naturopathy are:

1. The cause of disease is the accumulation of unnecessary wastes, which, if not properly eliminated, cause poison retention.
2. Your body is always striving for the ultimate good of the individual. Listen to its signals.
3. Given the proper environment, your body has the power to heal itself and to return to its normal stasis.

Naturopathic Practices

By way of review, a Naturopath works with you to restore and support your body's optimum health by using a variety of modalities including:

- Diet
- Herbs
- Exercise
- Rest
- Massage
- Recommendations for clients to seek harmony of body, mind, and spirit

The essentials of natural health can be grouped and evaluated in several ways. For the purpose of this book, we will look at them as ten key sections, divided into three categories. The categories and sections are:

Category 1: Basic Nutrients

- Air
- Water
- Sunlight
- Magnetic Field
- Food and Diet

Category 2: Physical Activity

- Exercise
- Rest

Category 3: Mental and Spiritual Health

- The Mind
- The Spirit
- Moderation and Balance

Naturopathic consultations are designed to help the client better understand the dietary and lifestyle factors that contribute to their specific and general health concerns. Documented recommendations help the client develop short and long-term **personalized** health strategies. They help facilitate practical, realistic transitions to dietary and lifestyle changes for improved health.

How To Use This Book

It is best to read through each section of this book at an unhurried pace, instead of reading it as you would a short story. You will find that most of the principles represent a "return to basics" approach, while the guidelines are presented in concentrated form. It may take several readings and reflection to appreciate the content and practical aspects of these principles and to develop your own health philosophy and strategy. The bibliography is a selected list of the many reputable works referred to in this book, and it should be consulted for further information and explanation. The appendices offer further guidelines on key topics. Also included is a Health Quotient (HQ) that you can use to evaluate your "Health IQ" according to the principles outlined in this book. I hope you will be encouraged in your reading and evaluate and reflect upon your personal health practices and strategies with an eye toward taking personal responsibility for owning and optimizing your total health. Once you have established a base, you may entertain other reinforcing practices beyond this book. The compact nature of this book in no way minimizes the importance of the information provided here, the depth and scope of which may surprise you. Careful concentration on the underlying principles and further review of the bibliographical material will affirm these points.

Finally, be critical of this book's content. Please provide any feedback regarding additions, deletions, or other modifications that would improve your understanding of its content and usefulness for future editions. Suggestions in the past from many health professionals, clients, health partners, friends and family proved valuable in the formation of this version and your recommendations could serve to improve the next version.

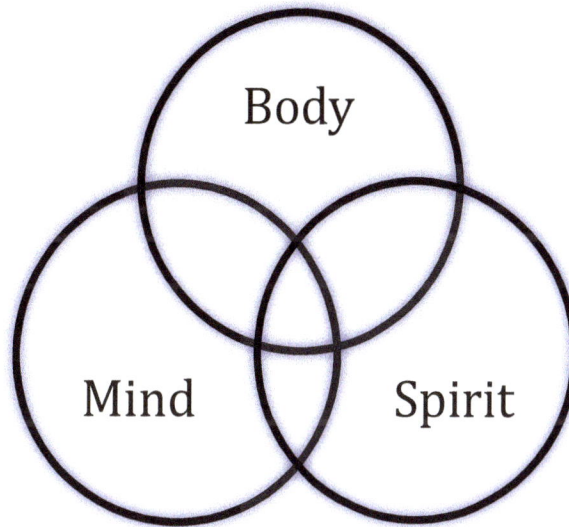

Total Health

Health is the harmonious integration of body, mind, and spirit. When all three elements are balanced and in harmony, we experience total health. These three components complement each other to the point that improved health in any one element improves the function of the remaining two elements, leading to total health of the person. Blockages in any one of these elements will, therefore, affect our *total health*.

With the harmonious integration of body, mind and spirit, we become resistant to the disorganized, disoriented, or diseased state. The following guidelines and principles offer a guide for demonstrating how to achieve optimum health in each component, leading to a state of harmonious integration, or total health.

ॐ • ॐ

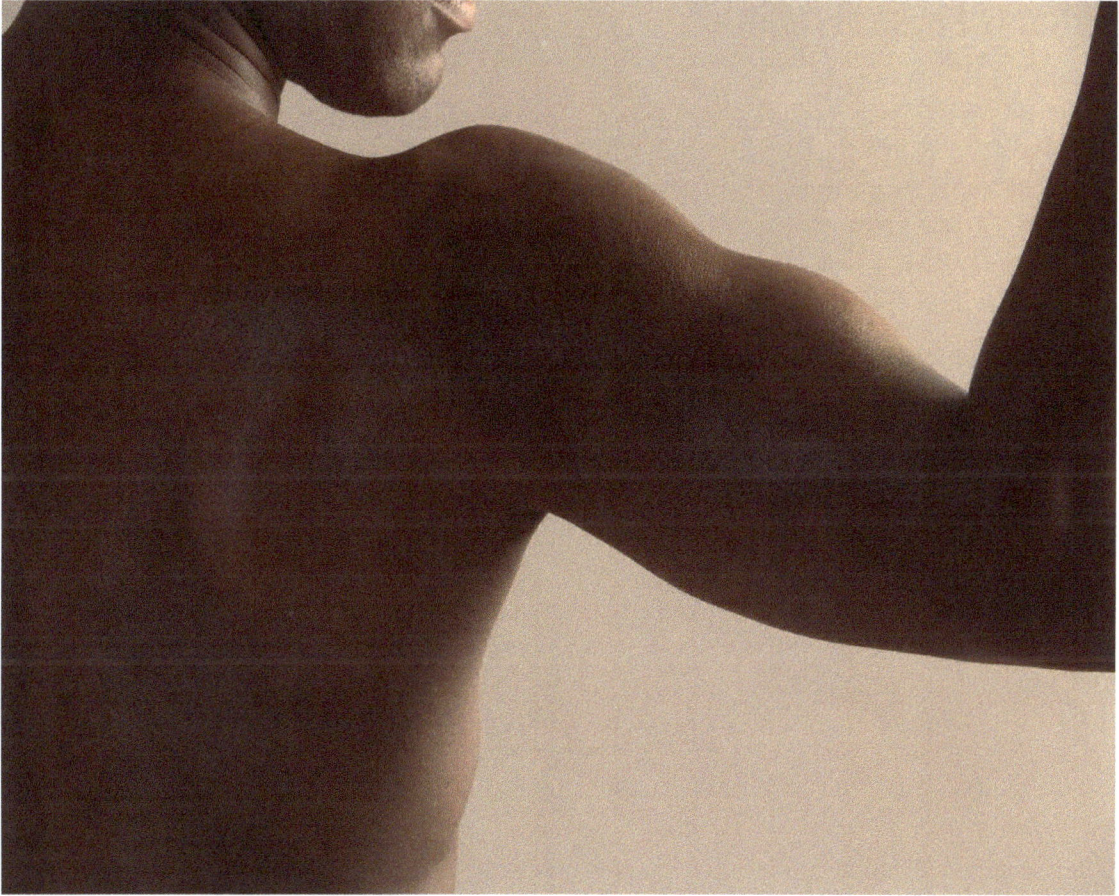

The Body

The body is the first and most logical place to begin. It is the medium through which the mind and spirit are maintained and developed for the improvement of personal character. Without your body, your mind and spirit cannot exist.

We will spend the most time looking at guidelines for the physical health of the body, not because it is the most important factor; but because human existence is most precarious without it,. Anything that nourishes the body nourishes and supports the brain, the nerves, the mind, and all vital aspects of our being.

Conversely, anything that stresses and harms the body will compromise the attainment of total health.

What is Physical Health?

Physical health is realized when we experience the full functional integrity of our bodies. It is a state of well-being where we experience physical vitality, freedom from disease, emotional balance, and clarity of mind and intellect. We experience functional integrity of our physiological systems and metabolic processes. Simply stated, everything is functioning the way it should.

A Formula for Physical Health

A simple formula for maintaining physical health is to maximize the nourishment of your body and eliminate accumulated waste, resulting in metabolic balance. This formula is the underlying basis for the experience of health. Health requires a healthy lifestyle. As we honor the basic laws of health through healthy lifestyle factors, we enjoy optimum physical health.

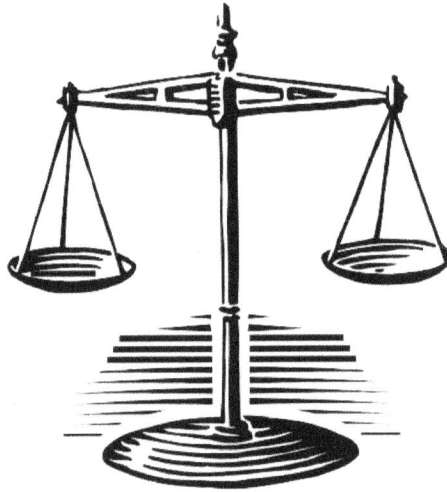

Maintaining Metabolic Balance
Maximizing Nourishment and Eliminating Waste

We will review the factors of maintaining physical health in the next section and examine elimination of accumulated toxins later in this book.

The Health Continuum

For each individual, health exists on a continuum from wellness to illness. Let's look at the health continuum, with some general definitions of the various levels of health and how they relate to the general population.

Health Continuum (View 1)

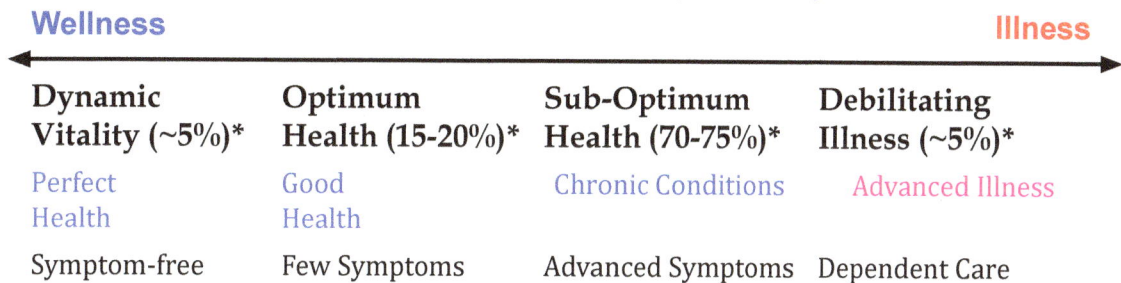

Wellness ←————————————————————————————→ **Illness**

Dynamic Vitality (~5%)*	Optimum Health (15-20%)*	Sub-Optimum Health (70-75%)*	Debilitating Illness (~5%)*
Perfect Health	Good Health	Chronic Conditions	Advanced Illness
Symptom-free	Few Symptoms	Advanced Symptoms	Dependent Care

*Percentage of people who are in this category

Health Continuum (View 2)

DYNAMIC VITALITY   (5-10%)

- Dynamic Vitality
- Harmonious Integration of Body/Mind/Spirit

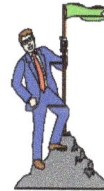

OPTIMUM HEALTH   (15-20%)

- General Sense of Wellness
- Biochemical and Bioenergetic Balance

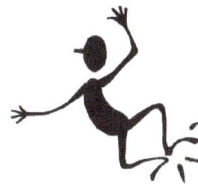

SUB-OPTIMUM HEALTH   (70-75%)

- Degenerative Conditions
- Walking Sick

DEBILITATING ILLNESS   (15-20%)

- Advanced Degeneration
- Disabling Illness

Explanation of the Health Continuum

Dynamic Vitality

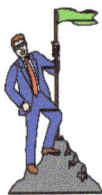

This category, which comprises approximately 5 percent of the American population, represents those who are genetically well endowed and tend to be more resilient to compromises in diet and lifestyle. They rarely get sick, tend to recover more easily from sickness, and tend to live long and fairly productive lives in spite of their diet and lifestyle. The basic principles of natural health will generally enhance the quality of life of persons in this category.

Optimum Health

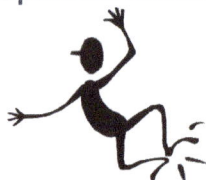

Experienced by 15–20 percent of the population, this category represents those who are generally in good health and are usually pursuing good dietary and lifestyle habits. This group lives long and productive lives primarily due to their application of the basic principles of natural health.

Sub-optimum Health

This is the largest group, representing 70–75 percent of the population. This category represents those who are experiencing any of a long list of chronic degenerative conditions including allergies, asthma, AIDS, headaches, PMS, fibroids, cancer, digestive conditions, skin conditions, obesity, arthritis, high blood pressure, diabetes, and over a hundred primary and secondary conditions.

Debilitating Illness

Like the first group, the first group comprises approximately 5 percent of the population and represents those with serious illnesses including advanced degenerative conditions, structural problems and genetic deficiencies. This group is generally bedridden and/or experiencing major compromises in their function and performance.

Diet and lifestyle factors (lifestyle medicine) have the greatest impact and exert the most influence in the first three categories of the health continuum. They play more of a complementary role in the last category where traditional medicine protocols are generally the most effective and may even be necessary. Traditional medicine, in the form of prescription drugs and antibiotic drugs, is the primary approach for many in the last two categories. It should be used only when necessary for the third category but is generally the most effective for the last category.

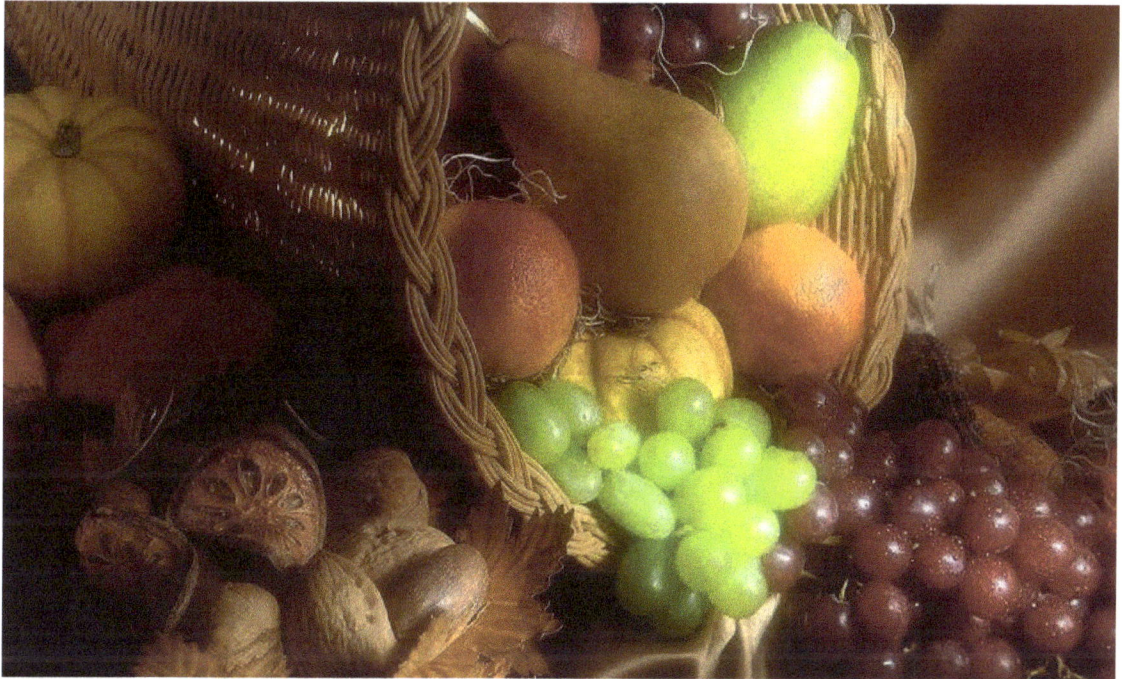

The Hierarchy
of Nutrients

A Unique Perspective on Diet

The purpose of this section is to present a unique and simple way of looking at nutrition as it relates to experiencing a healthy lifestyle. This unique model is The Hierarchy of Nutrients. A hierarchy is a set of groups classified according to their level of importance. This offers an approach to categorizing foods and nutrients with the most integrity to those with the least integrity as they relate to maximizing nourishment. This is a simple yet powerful way of showing how foods affect health and vitality. As a naturopath, I emphasize looking to nature as the provider for both nourishment and healing of the human body. This hierarchy categorizes nutrients in a way that exposes many popular misconceptions about foods and empowers you to make the best choices from available nutritional options.

The Hierarchy of Nutrients

The guiding principles underlying the nutrient hierarchy are as follows:

- God, through nature, placed us on this planet to thrive and not just to survive.
- This planet provides the nutrients we need most in the highest quantity.
- This planet provides the nutrients we need most in the most easily available form.

So, let's look at our nutritional requirements from this alternative, and perhaps new, perspective which categorizes all nutrients into five food groups.

Nutrient Hierarchy

HIGHEST QUALITY NUTRIENTS most important nutrients		LOWEST QUALITY NUTRIENTS least important nutrients		
Group 1 Basic Nutrients	Group 2 Natural Raw Foods	Group 3 Grains & Legumes	Group 4 Flesh Foods Dairy Products	Group 5 Refined & Processed Foods
Air Water Sunlight Earth's Magnetic Field	Fruits Vegetables Nuts & Seeds	Wheat, Corn, Oats, Rye, Barley, etc. Beans, Peas, etc.	Beef, Pork, Poultry & Fish Milk & Cheese	Processed Foods Synthetic Foods
Hierarchy of Nutrients			Standard American Diet	

Figure 1. Hierarchy of Nutrients

The basic formula for explaining the nutrient hierarchy is this: God provides for us, through nature, all the nutrients we need to thrive and not just to survive. Furthermore, the nutrients we need most are provided most abundantly and in the most easily available form. So, let's look at physical nourishment from this alternative and perhaps new, perspective. According to this new perspective on nourishment, the nutrient sources have been divided into five nutritive groups.

Nutrient Group 1: Basic Nutrients

The first four nutrients are the most basic (foundational) nutrients for all life forms on this planet. They are so abundant and available that we generally take them for granted without realizing their significance to experiencing high vitality and optimum health. The nutrients in this category are air, water, sunlight and the earth. We can live without food for several months, but a lack of the basic nutrients in Group 1 will severely impact general health and well-being after just a short period of deficiency. Let's take a brief look at each of these from a nutritious standpoint.

Air

Air is the most important nutrient since as little as 3–5 minutes of deprivation will have very apparent and serious effects on our health and our very existence. Every cell in our body needs life-giving oxygen. High-quality fresh air is actually electrified. The oxygen molecule is negatively charged or "negatively ionized." This negatively charged oxygen gives rise to a number of benefits, including:

- Improved functioning of the lungs
- Improved relaxation and ability to deal with stress
- Improved mental clarity
- Improved healing of wounds
- Decreased survival of bacteria and viruses
- Stimulated appetite and easier digestion
- Induced sound and restful sleep

We will show how this important nutrient is related to our ideal diet as we continue our evaluation of the nutrient hierarchy. Clearly, air is the first and most important nutrient and it behooves all of us to get as much fresh air as possible.

Water

The planet is 70–75 percent water and our bodies are 70–75 percent water. We can live without water for perhaps a week or two at the most. The consequences of a deficiency of water are very well understood, and the body's need for water is already appreciated by many. A wealth of information has been published on the subject of water and its impact on a variety of disease states. This research implies that adequate water combined with other aspects of a healthful lifestyle may help postpone or prevent a variety of diseases and their complications. Some important factors relating to water include the following. Water does the following:Thins and increases the blood volume

- Acts as a natural diuretic
- Helps eliminate accumulated waste from your body
- Manages body temperature during exercise
- Acts as the universal solvent
- Aids in digestion, assimilation, and elimination of nutrients.

Sunlight

Sunlight supports all life and is necessary for the synthesis of all plant nutrients. We can live without sunlight for extended periods of time, longer than without air and water, but not without serious consequences. Excessive ultraviolet light from the sun can indeed increase the risk of skin cancer and cataracts, but judicious amounts of sunlight can be extremely beneficial. For example, sunshine plays a critical role in helping to prevent osteoporosis. Some of the important benefits of sunlight include the following:

- Converts cholesterol into vitamin D, an essential factor in maintaining good bone health. As little as 15 minutes of exposure provides minimum requirements for vitamin D
- Improves vitamin and mineral absorption
- Stores energy in muscles and nerves
- Improves overall metabolic function and efficiency
- Boosts the immune response that kills bacteria and viruses
- Controls the chemistry of the blood
- Increases a sense of well-being and energizes the personality.

Earth

It may seem strange to classify the earth as a nutrient. The earth, however, plays the following two important roles in the context of nutrients:

1. An electromagnetic field emanates from the earth.
2. The earth produces our food.

The Earth is a large magnet with a North and a South pole; it has a metallic core, and it spins and emits a low-grade magnetic field. This magnetic field provides several health benefits, including improved immune function, energy, bone density, brain and nerve function. Like sunlight, an electromagnetic field deficiency can be endured longer than a deficiency of air and water. Still we have learned quite a bit from the experiences of astronauts traveling in outer space about the serious consequences of decreased gravity and long-term deficiencies of the Earth's electromagnetic field.

The most obvious benefit of the earth is the nutrients it provides in various forms for the nourishment and optimum performance of our metabolic and systemic functions.

Now, as discussed above, let's connect the basic nutrients in Nutrient Group 1 to all other nutrient intakes. The relationship between these basic nutrients in Group 1 and all the remaining Nutrient Groups is that all the remaining nutrients are categorized based on the way in which they manifest and present the other basic, life-giving nutrients.

Nutrient Group 2: Natural Raw Foods

Natural raw foods – fruits, vegetables, nuts and seeds–are the second category of essential foods. These foods are abundantly supplied by the earth and require very little human effort to be produced. They are already in the most efficient form for human consumption. All can be eaten in their natural, raw form without preparation of any kind. Nutrient Group 2 foods all contain the basic nutrients found in Nutrient Group 1 and provide them to the body in their most bio-available and integrated form. An added benefit is that the leaves of trees provide all our breathable air; trees are the lungs of this planet.

In many respects, fruit is the most efficient and nourishing of all foods. It can be thought of as a cocktail of air, water, sunlight and the earth's nutrient resources. Key characteristics of fruit (and to a lesser extent the remaining foods in this category) include the following. Fruits:

Are higher in water content than other foods.

- Have sunlight locked into every atom.
- Grow on trees whose roots reach down to absorb both the Earth's electromagnetic field and the Earth's micronutrients--minerals and other plant nutrients.
- All the foods in this category can be eaten in their natural, raw form with no preparation required.

Plants, with the aid of microorganisms and an adequate supply of basic soil nutrients, have the ability to synthesize minerals and other nutrients. They, effectively, can "eat" soil. Minerals and other absorbed or plant-synthesized nutrients are then organized into fruits, vegetables, seeds, and nuts for optimum human consumption and assimilation.

Nutrient Group 3: Grains and Legumes

While the general view is that grains and legumes (beans and peas) are the foundational foods of a health-producing diet, it should be noted that all these foods generally require some form of preparation prior to consumption. In addition, they are not as hydrated as the natural, raw foods in Nutrient Group 2 and should be eaten in moderation. Their clear value is that they contain a high concentration of nutrients (primarily complex carbohydrates and proteins) and can be stored for long periods of time in the event of flood, famine, warfare, or other factors affecting the availability of natural raw foods noted in the previous group.

Nutrient Group 4: Flesh Foods and Dairy Products

Flesh foods, which include fish, meat, poultry, and dairy products, are surprisingly low on the nutrient hierarchy. These foods provide the most concentrated nutrients (primarily fats and proteins), but they also place significant stress on our bodies. They are difficult to digest, are highly acidic and/or mucus-producing, and put a considerable strain on the gastrointestinal tract and liver in breaking them down for assimilation and on the kidneys for elimination from the body. When we eat flesh foods we are receiving our plant-based nutrients second-hand. The commercial production of flesh foods, along with the compromised environments and conditions they are exposed to, further impacts the integrity of this food source. The liberal use of growth hormones, antibiotics, genetically engineered feed and exposure to other environmental hazards and conditions, make consumption of flesh foods significantly more problematic than fifty to one hundred years ago.

There is much misinformation and many misconceptions about flesh foods and dairy products, primarily due to brilliant marketing, rather than valid scientific evaluation. These foods should be eaten in very limited quantities, if at all.

Nutrient Group 5: Refined and Processed Foods

All of the previous categories of foods and nutrients come from nature. Processed and refined foods, however, are not provided by nature. They are made by the food industry and are really junk foods. These include most of the foods that come in boxes, plastic containers, or cans, and they generally contain preservatives, additives, stabilizers, dyes, colorings, artificial flavoring and other nutritive-compromising ingredients. Plant analogues, refined sugar, food isolates, isolated vitamins and minerals, synthetic drugs and even poorly cooked foods, all belong in this category. They are low in essential nutrients and/or leach essential nutrients from your body.

03 • 80

For centuries, our planet provided
all the essentials for human nourishment.
No company can improve upon the
integrity of naturally produced, planet-
based foods.

Relationship of Health to the Hierarchy of Nutrients

Those individuals who experience higher levels of health tend to utilize the higher Nutrient Groups in the Hierarchy of Nutrients. Conversely, those experiencing poor health and illness at the lower end of the health continuum tend to get a disproportionate amount of their nourishment from the lower Nutrient Groups in the Hierarchy of Nutrients. As a naturopath, I spend considerable time evaluating each individual's dietary factors as they relate to their degenerative conditions. I encourage those individuals at the lower end of the Hierarchy of Nutrients to consider dietary modifications that include appropriate foods from the upper end of the Hierarchy of Nutrients. The amount and concentration of the foods are evaluated based on each individual's requirements and capacities.

The Hierarchy of Nutrients is not a cure-all for all conditions. As a naturopath, I recommend that my clients consider additional lifestyle factors, including exercise and rest, stress management, prayer and meditation, and other important natural remedies. I also understand pharmaceutical and surgical approaches important role,, especially in acute conditions.

Diet and lifestyle factors have a long-term record of producing the best results for most chronic degenerative conditions. Applying the dietary principles inherent in the Hierarchy of Nutrients, based on an individual's requirements and capacities, with the appropriate application of lifestyle factors, is the most effective approach for experiencing optimum, radiant health. From a nutrient standpoint, the aim is to move as high on the Hierarchy of Nutrients scale as required for meeting your desired health goals.

Health is a precious gift, and most people can experience major improvements in their health by making the best choices from the options available. This requires some personal effort on your part and will generally require working with health professionals and educators for guidance in this lifestyle change endeavor. This unique perspective on evaluating food choices is provided to help you in the exciting endeavor of taking charge of your life and achieving your goal of health and happiness. The choice is yours.

The following graphic comparison summarizes the relationship of the Hierarchy of Nutrients to the Health Continuum, discussed at the beginning of this section.

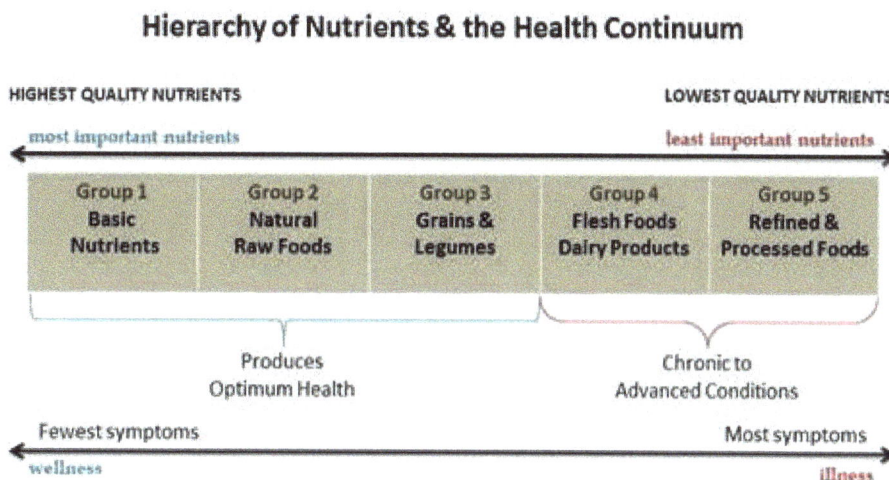

Hierarchy of Nutrients & the Health Continuum

HIGHEST QUALITY NUTRIENTS			LOWEST QUALITY NUTRIENTS	
most important nutrients			least important nutrients	
Group 1 Basic Nutrients	Group 2 Natural Raw Foods	Group 3 Grains & Legumes	Group 4 Flesh Foods Dairy Products	Group 5 Refined & Processed Foods

Produces
Optimum Health

Chronic to
Advanced Conditions

Fewest symptoms   Most symptoms

wellness   illness

Figure 2. Hierarchy of Nutrients and the Health Continuum

Now, let's look at Nutrient Group 1 in more detail. This group consists of Air, Water, Sunlight, and the Earth's Magnetic field. Some of the material in the next section has been adapted from "Fill your life with Celebrations," a presentation series and publication of the General Conference of the Seventh-day Adventist Church.

Air

Air is so abundant and immediately available that we tend to take it for granted.

Air is the most important nutrient. This is obvious because as little as three minutes of deprivation will have very apparent and serious effects on our health and our very existence.

Air is the first essential of a healthy body. We can live without food for several months and without water for several days; but we cannot live without air for more than just a few minutes. Pure, fresh air oxygenates and enlivens your body. Impure air is one of the greatest causes of poor health.

One of the important functions of air is providing oxygen for combustion (metabolism) of ingested nutrients and burning waste products that are constantly forming in your body. When the supply of oxygen is diminished, waste and poisons can accumulate. Any treatment that does not encourage the use of good, clean, and fresh air will be significantly compromised in its effectiveness.

Pure, natural air has been sterilized by the rays of the sun. It is also washed by the rain and purified by the synergistic action of plant life. With the disappearance of many of our forests and the effects of industrially generated pollutants, our supply of fresh, pure air is almost nonexistent in our day-to-day living and working environments. Health-conscious people should be knowledgeable about their environments and the quality of the air they breathe.

Air quality tends to be best in the early morning and late evening. The best supply of clean, fresh air can be found in the mountains, in large wooded areas, near large bodies of water, and in some remote places far from industry and automobiles. Clean, fresh air is negatively charged, and polluted air is positively charged. Air pollution abounds with tobacco smoke, automobile emissions, industrial wastes, burning grasslands, etc. When indoor air is poor, a negative ion generator can be used to improve air quality. However, there is no real substitute for fresh, clean outdoor air.

Because fresh air is important to health, efforts need to be made to breathe natural clean air, for example during outdoor morning exercise. A vitality will thus be imparted that is superior to that achieved in stale, recirculated air or that found in smoky rooms, congested offices, or noisy factories. The reporting of discomfort and symptoms related to office environments have led to such terms as sick-building syndrome. This is particularly noted in sealed buildings with centrally controlled mechanical ventilation. Associated conditions include allergies, infections, Legionnaire's disease, and worsening of asthma because of air-borne irritants. This highlights the importance of breathing fresh, clean air.

Breathing is a natural spontaneous automatic activity, taking in and moving a total of approximately 20,000 liters of air daily. As the lungs inhale the air oxygen and carbon dioxide exchange in more than 600 million air sacs, called the alveoli. These alveoli are lined by a network of fine capillaries containing blood.

Air and blood are separated by these thin walls, which are only two cells thick. Here, the exchange of gases by diffusion occurs. Blood that is low in oxygen, full of carbon dioxide, is brought to the lungs so carbon dioxide may be released and oxygen is taken up. Many millions of red blood cells then carry the oxygen-rich blood to nourish all the body's tissues and cells. This exchange of oxygen and carbon dioxide is completed within milliseconds, and it takes about one minute for a complete circuit of the body!

Important Qualities of Air

1. Air is a food. In fact, it is more essential than any other food and must be used for the performance of many vital functions. The oxygen in air is carried by the blood to every cell in the body and essential for cellular metabolism.
2. Air contains electricity. Fresh air charges your nerves and muscles with electricity and increases your energy.
3. Air is a healing agent. A wound will not heal without air. It acts as both a purifier and a deodorizer.
4. Fresh air acts as an agent in producing a more positive attitude. It strengthens and nourishes the nervous system. Foul air is depressing and stressful to your body.
5. The oxygen source in air is replenished by the leaves of trees. We, in turn, breathe out carbon dioxide, an essential nutrient for plants! God created this synergistic cycle so that we would always have fresh supplies of oxygen to maintain optimum health.

Daily exposure to fresh air is very important for vibrant health. Each day you should begin with an air bath. Exposing your body to the air with as little clothing as is practical can be very refreshing and revitalizing for your entire body.

Basic deep breathing can be incorporated into your daily routine. All bodily functions, including proper digestion, need clean air, and proper breathing aids assimilation and metabolism. Most people tend to breathe significantly less than their true capacity. Deep breathing, which starts in the diaphragm, is extremely important to physical health. Some basic principles of deep breathing are discussed in a later section of this book.

The lungs are a major organ of elimination. Shallow breathing limits the elimination of carbon dioxide and other harmful gases through your lungs. Your breathing should be relaxed and done within your capacity. Breathing in (inhalation) energizes your body and breathing out (exhalation) relaxes the body. When using breathing exercises, it is important that your exhalation is at least as long as your inhalation and most authorities recommend that it be slightly longer.

Most aerobic activities encourage deep breathing and promote functional integrity of the respiratory system. Certain disciplines like yoga, martial arts, and several holistic techniques encourage deep, controlled, and health-promoting breathing. This is our simplest and most important bodily function for sustaining ourselves.

Air is so important and necessary that we cannot even commit suicide by just stopping our breath. If we hold our breath to the point of blacking out, our brainstem automatically takes over and causes us to start breathing again.

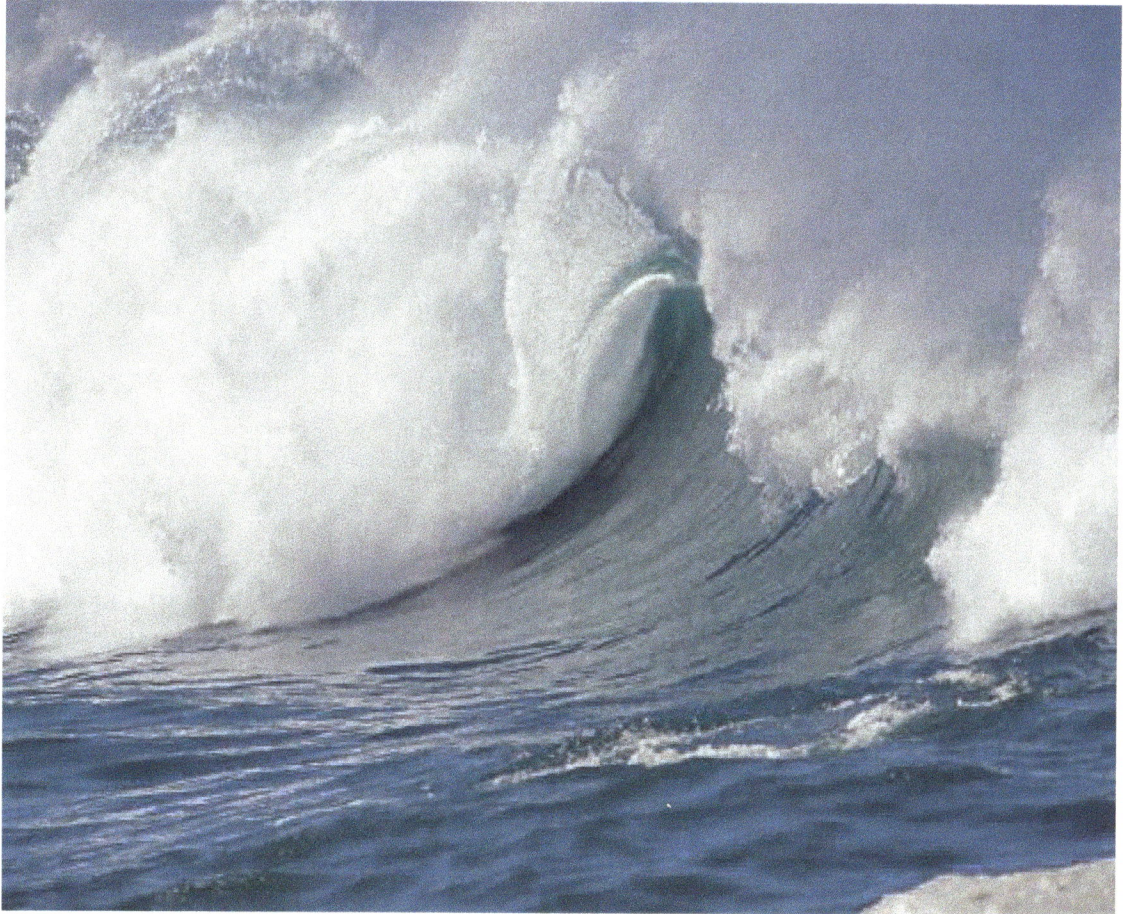

Water

The planet is 70–75% water and so are our bodies–we are a template of the planet.

The most precious of all liquids is water. Our earth is more than two-thirds water; however, most of it is unsuitable for agriculture and human consumption. Therefore, water is a precious resource and its conservation is important. It is indispensable for optimum health.

We can live without water for perhaps a week or two at the most, and deficiencies in this area are very well understood and appreciated. The planet is 70–75 percent water, like our bodies, demonstrating that we are in close concert with the planet, insofar as water is concerned. This illustrates the workings of the formula of abundance and availability noted earlier in the Hierarchy of Nutrients.

By weight a newborn infant is approximately 75 percent water, and an adult is approximately 70 percent water. A 150-pound man has approximately 105 pounds of water in his body. Water is essential for the function of every cell of the body. Almost every cell and tissue of our body contains water, is continually bathed in fluid, and requires water to perform its functions!

All the body's tissues, vital fluids, and secretions contain water. The brain's gray matter is approximately 85 percent water, blood is approximately 83 percent water, muscles are approximately 75 percent water, and even hard, marrow bones are 20–25 percent water. All major processes in the body, including circulation, digestion, and elimination, require the presence of water. Since the water supply is not recycled and we are losing it constantly, it must be replenished constantly.

Water is imperative to maintaining and regaining health. When water is used improperly it results in sickness and disease. Natural, pure water is the best source of water. The compromised quality of most water supplies, which includes pollution, toxic waste, and forced chlorination, generally causes alternate supplies of water to be required. Health-conscious people should be knowledgeable about their environment and the quality of the water they use.

Water pollution abounds because of contamination by sewage pumped into rivers and oceans; runoff from garbage dumps; oil spills; industrial wastes such as mercury, lead, and polychlorinated biphenyls (PCBs); chemical fertilizers and pesticide residues; and so forth. Filtered or bottled water are often the most practical way to consume optimum water. Distilled water provides the best results for most purposes, especially for cleansing and fasting programs.

Your body requires approximately 64–80 ounces, or 8–10 eight-ounce glasses of water a day. A general rule is one ounce for every two pounds of body weight, modified to meet special circumstances like activity level, outside temperature, and health status. It is important to ensure adequate water intake to maintain bodily functions including making good blood, feeding the cells, oxidation of the cells, waste elimination, and regulating the temperature of your body.

Living a natural lifestyle and eating a natural diet consisting primarily of fruits and vegetables seldom generates thirst. Fruits and vegetables are high water-content foods (more than 70 percent water); therefore, there may be little need to drink additional water. The recommendation of 8–10 glasses a day is for a cooked-food oriented diet. Water from fruits and vegetables is distilled by the synergistic action of the sun on them and provides pure, clean, thirst-quenching and life-giving water.

Most animals in the wild live on fruits and vegetables and drink very modest amounts of water. Humans, by nature, also require only modest amounts of drinking water. Nature's supply of water is best provided through natural foods, which are composed mainly of water. Fruits and vegetables act as nature's water filters. The water content of food is altered by excessive cooking which also compromises the water content.

When unnatural foods are taken into the body, nature tries to counteract the accumulated waste by diluting them. This in turn causes thirst, which explains the great thirst of many people. Satisfying this thirst with the introduction of large quantities of unnatural fluids can be very distressful and harmful to the optimum performance of our bodies. Over-consumption of fluid, even water, causes several problems including bloating, excessive water retention, distention of blood vessels and organs, and other harmful results.

Drinking water in excess can have harmful effects on your body. Just as we should not eat when we're not hungry, we should not drink when we're not thirsty. Drinking excessively can interfere with the normal function of the body. It can also overtax the kidneys and cause excessive urination. Eating an adequate amount of live, fresh fruits and vegetables supplies an abundance of the purest naturally distilled water that is full of fragrance, organic minerals, and life-giving nutrients.

When required, water is best taken between meals and should be sipped, not gulped down. It should be at room temperature or warmed for best results. Iced water, in particular, can be very harmful to the internal organs, especially the kidneys. It tends to shock and put the internal organs into spasm. Digestion is stopped until the water can be warmed to body temperature, thereby delaying or causing incomplete food breakdown.

Water is also beneficial externally. It can be used to reduce the heat of the body in cases of fever, increase the heat of the body in cases of low vitality, cleanse the skin and tonify your body.

Hydrotherapy, properly administered colonics, contrast footbaths and showers and steam baths are some of the external uses of water that promote and maintain health. In hydrotherapy, hot and cold treatments are applied for improved nourishment, muscle relaxation, stimulation, and circulation. Colon hydrotherapy uses warm water to gently clean out and stimulate reflex points in the colon. Contrast showers and foot baths, which employ alternating hot and cold water, improve circulation and strengthen the immune system. Steam baths open and cleanse the pores of the skin.

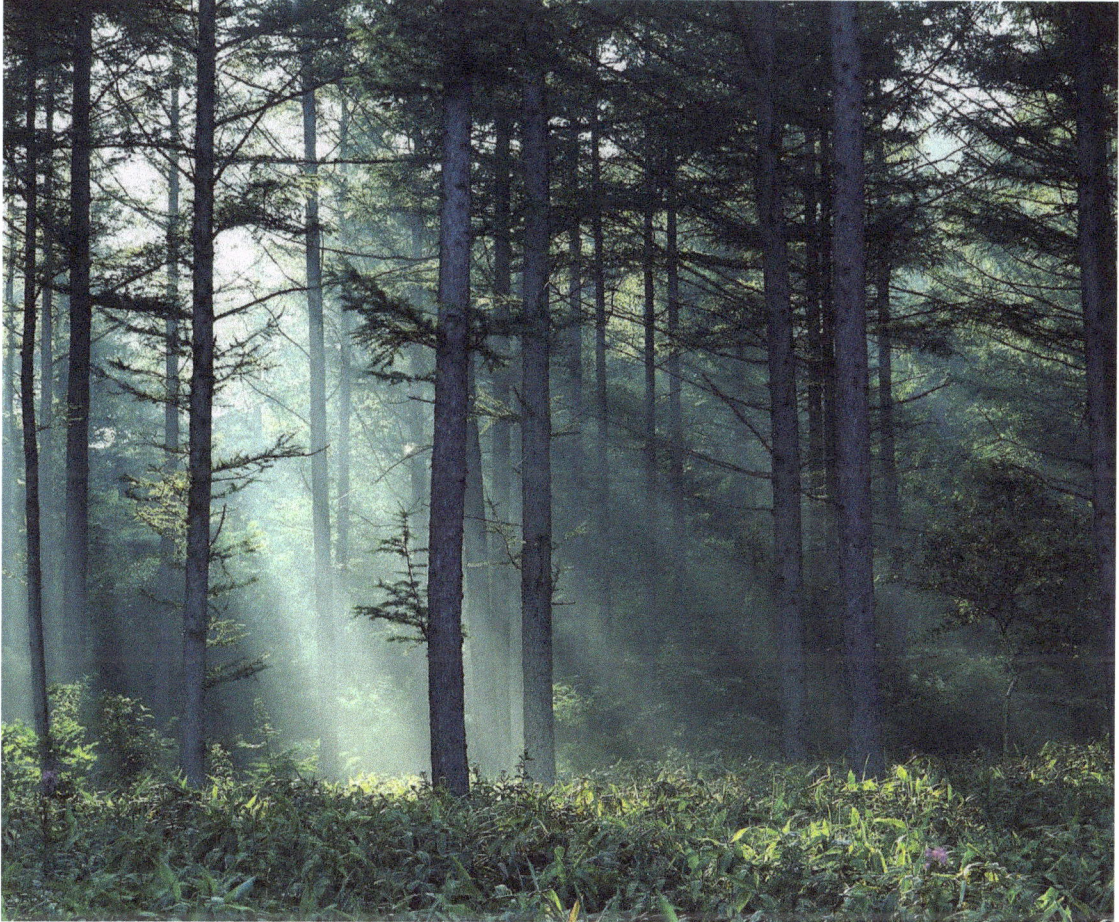

Sunlight

Sunlight is locked in the atoms of all plants that grow on the earth.

We can live without sunlight for extended periods of time, longer than both air and water, but not without serious consequences. All life on earth depends on the energy of the sun. In short, life would cease if there was no sunshine.

Sunlight is composed of many different energy levels, transmitted in the form of electromagnetic waves. The rays of the sun expose humankind to three types of light in different wavelengths:

1. Invisible light - Ultraviolet light provides the majority of the biological effects, both positive and negative, to humanity's health (5 percent of the solar radiation).
2. Infrared light provides warmth (54 percent of the solar emissions).
3. Visible light (40 percent of the solar radiation).
4. Shorter cosmic rays, gamma rays, X-rays, longer radio waves, and electromagnetic waves constitute the rest.

Some obvious benefits of the sun are vitamin D, improved vitamin and mineral absorption, and overall improvement in metabolic function and efficiency. Sunshine helps maintain ambient temperatures of the planet. In this way it supports both plant and animal existence and is a vital ingredient in our environment.

Sunlight aids in the availability of several nutrients including vitamin D, cholesterol management and calcium assimilation. In addition to the known nutrient-giving properties of the sun, there are many complex and even unknown benefits. The abundant energy and life-giving properties available from sunlight to the plant kingdom have similar positive effects on humans who eat those plants.

Daily sunlight is required for all healthy, living things to develop, grow, and flourish. As little as 20 minutes of exposure a day will have powerful, positive effects on your body. The full-spectrum light and energy provided by the sun supports visual integrity and supplies the subtle, vibratory energy underlying all plant and human function. Overexposure should be avoided at all times, especially to midday sun in the summer months.

Insufficient sunshine results in a pale complexion, lowered physical vitality, and poor health. Exposure to the sun results in a healthy-looking complexion, energized blood, and overall good health. Sunshine is both a natural and effective healing agent.

Important Effects of the Sun

Sunshine can have the following effects on your body:

1. Chemical. It unlocks the vitamins in your food. The process of digestion is incomplete without sunshine. The more light and heat we receive from the sun, the less heavy food we require. Sunlight in effect controls the chemistry of the blood.
2. Physical. It warms your body and at the same time energizes it. Sunshine helps and encourages every important function of the body. When the sun shines on your skin it quickly stores a tremendous amount of energy in your body. The nerve endings absorb the vibrant energy and transmit this energy to your entire nervous system.
3. Psychological. Exposure to sunshine offers you the experience of peace, joy, happiness, and a feeling of relief and freedom. Your mind immediately senses that your body is in its natural medium and your thoughts begin to take on a loftier aspect.

Eating in sunlight, when practical, enhances digestion and encourages a natural diet. A healthy, natural diet, in turn, enhances interest and tolerance of sunlight. If your body has the right nutrients, it will respond very favorably to sunlight.

In modern times, we notice a decline in the interest in sunshine. Until a few years ago, the general public ignored the marvelous health-giving power of sunlight and was familiar only to a handful of people. Now there seems to be an awakening of the wonderful beneficial effects of the sun's rays for the health and vitality of the human body. Several bacteria and germs cannot live in direct sunlight and many diseases are curable by allowing the sun to come in direct contact with your body for various periods of time.

Natural sunlight contains the full spectrum of colors, which provides the best medium for visual acuity. The underlying energy systems of your body are constantly feeding on and storing up the life-giving elements from the rays of the sun. Sunshine, like air, acts as a stimulant, tonic, and healer.

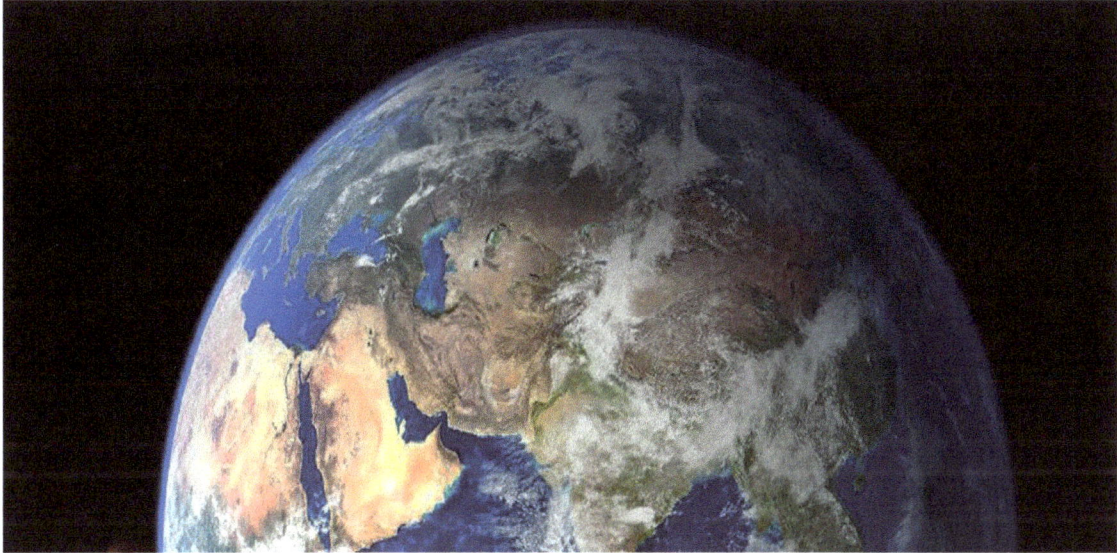

Magnetic Field of the Earth

The earth is a large magnet with a metallic core, which spins and generates a magnetic field.

Like sunlight, the need for a magnetic field can be compromised longer than air and water. Still, we have learned quite a bit, especially from the experiences of astronauts traveling in outer space, about the serious consequences of long-term deficiencies in the Earth's magnetic field. The earth, a large magnet with a North and South Pole, has a metallic core, which spins and emits a low-grade magnetic field.

The importance of the earth's magnetic field is receiving more attention. Along with air, water and sunlight, the earth's magnetic field rounds out the fourth element required for all basic life functions on this planet. If any of these factors are sufficiently compromised or eliminated, all life as we know it would cease to exist on this planet. Our bodies are designed for optimum performance in a synergistic cocoon of oxygen-saturated air, naturally mineralized water, energizing sunlight, and a vitalizing magnetic field. While all these elements are required for balanced and optimal function of our bodily processes, the earth's magnetic field is probably the most overlooked element in evaluating and sustaining optimal health.

The earth's magnetic field is experienced in two primary forms. First of all, it is a component of all plant life. The elements of air, water, sunlight, and electromagnetic energy all work together for the growth and presentation of all vegetation. The roots of all plant life can be thought of as an umbilical cord connecting them to the earth. Accordingly, the planet's pervasive life-giving nutrients – air, water, sunlight, and the Earth's magnetic field nurture all plant life. Once this umbilical cord is cut, i.e., removed from its connection to the earth, this synergistic nurturing aspect is broken. This is a major reason why eating fresh, unrefined fruits, vegetables, nuts, seeds and other produce from our earth's bountiful supply provides the highest nutritional integrity.

Secondly, the earth's magnetic field is a natural component of our environment. Like air, water, and sunlight, it is a component of our atmosphere. This magnetic field affects the optimum function of our metabolic, hormonal, cerebrospinal, circulatory, nervous, and other vital body processes. When we walk barefoot on grass in a wooded and/or water-enriched environment, we experience a sense of peace, calm, and well-being resulting from the complementary flow of magnetic energy.

Unfortunately, like air, water, and sunlight, the earth's magnetic field has also been polluted and compromised over time. Metal in buildings (and sometimes in our bodies), paved roads, synthetic clothes and structures, electrical appliances, computers and a whole host of the "fruits of civilization" serve to compromise and cause a deficiency in our body's electromagnetic integrity. Some studies suggest that our earth's magnetic field has been reduced by as much as 50 percent over the past 500 to 1,000 years. Other sources indicate that we experience only 10 percent of the earth's magnetic field that existed 4,000 years ago. This deficiency offers some obvious implications for our ability to experience optimum health.

There is no substitute for anything produced by nature, whether it is air, water, sunlight, food, or electromagnetic energy. However, there are several opportunities for supplementing deficiencies in our traumatized environment. Poor air quality in our working or living environment can be supplemented with air purification ionizers, polluted water can be purified through various forms of filtration, and food can be supplemented with herbs and other vital foods that concentrate needed nutrients. Magnetic therapy, also referred to as biomagnetic therapy, can also be used to supplement our requirements for magnetic field energy.

Magnetic therapy is the application of specially designed magnets to the body for therapeutic purposes. They come in various strengths, from low intensity to high intensity (from below 1,000 gauss to over 12,000 gauss) and polarities (negative, positive and bipolar). Magnetic therapy is generally safe, non-invasive and non-toxic when used appropriately. Caution should be exercised in patients with pacemakers (although most low Gauss magnets do not affect newer pacemakers), metal devices inserted in the body, and in the first trimester of pregnancy. Most people usually respond positively to the use of magnetic health products, but individual requirements and capacities must be respected for optimum performance. With over 30 million people using magnetic health products worldwide, an impressive record of virtually no harmful side effects has been realized.

The healing power of magnets has been known for thousands of years. During the third century B.C., Aristotle was the first person in recorded history to speak about the therapeutic properties of magnets. Many other ancient cultures, including the Egyptian, Hebrew, Arabic, Chinese, and Indian had knowledge of and used magnets for healing purposes. In modern days, the experiences of astronauts returning from outer space with significant reduction in bone density and a wide variety of "space illnesses" has created a resurgence in the scientific community's acknowledgement of and focus on the importance of magnetic fields for optimal biological function and performance.

Magnets are available in a variety of convenient shapes and sizes that may be applied to an injury or pain site on the body. They can also be molded to be used as insoles for shoes and incorporated into a variety of devices such as bracelets, necklaces, mattress pads, pillow-like head supports, and joint and muscle supports. The magnets themselves are not responsible for the healing. They create an environment for our cells and body functions to operate more efficiently and they support our body's natural curative and restorative processes.

Magnets have been found to be especially effective in improving circulation, reducing (and often eliminating) joint and muscle pain, inflammation and significantly improving sleep and energy. Many degenerative processes, including asthma, arthritis, memory loss, gout, cancer, aids, high blood pressure and as much as 95 percent of the compromised conditions we experience tend to respond favorably when these factors are present.

Important Effects of Magnetic Energy

The following is a summary of some of the specific factors known to be involved in biomagnetic application, magnetic stimulation, and improvement in the body's electromagnetic integrity.

- Increased blood flow, resulting in increased oxygen and nutrient-carrying capacity, both of which are basic to supporting the body's natural healing processes.

- Stimulation of the migration of calcium, sodium, potassium and other ions is necessary for reducing pain and inflammation, and for proper functioning of the nervous system and other vital functions.

- Alteration of the pH balance of various body fluids, providing the proper acid/alkaline environment for certain body functions.

- Stimulation of enzymatic and hormone activity from the endocrine glands.

- Elimination or reduction of tumors because of improved cellular and immune function.

- Improvement in strength by as much as 20 percent.

- Improvement in chemistry, electrical nerve energy, and promotion of the health of every cell in the body.

Although relatively little research funding is made available in the United States in this area, magnetic therapy complements both conventional and alternative protocols. Diagnostic technologies, including magnetic resonance imaging (MRI), use intensities as high as 20,000 Gauss, which is significantly higher than most magnetic health and wellness products on the market. Several countries, including Japan, Russia, and Germany, use magnets as approved medical devices. Although proven and accepted for a wide variety of health issues worldwide, they are currently available in the United States primarily for self-help use.

Magnetic therapy should grow significantly with the increasing use and proven performance of several related energetic modalities such as acupuncture and acupressure, and increased public demand for low-cost, effective and noninvasive treatment for increasing health challenges. It can play an important role in the increasing emphasis on integrated medicine as practiced by forward-thinking physicians. Extensive research continues to take place outside of the United States, and it is simply a matter of time until the many important implications it offers for optimum health become available to the general public.

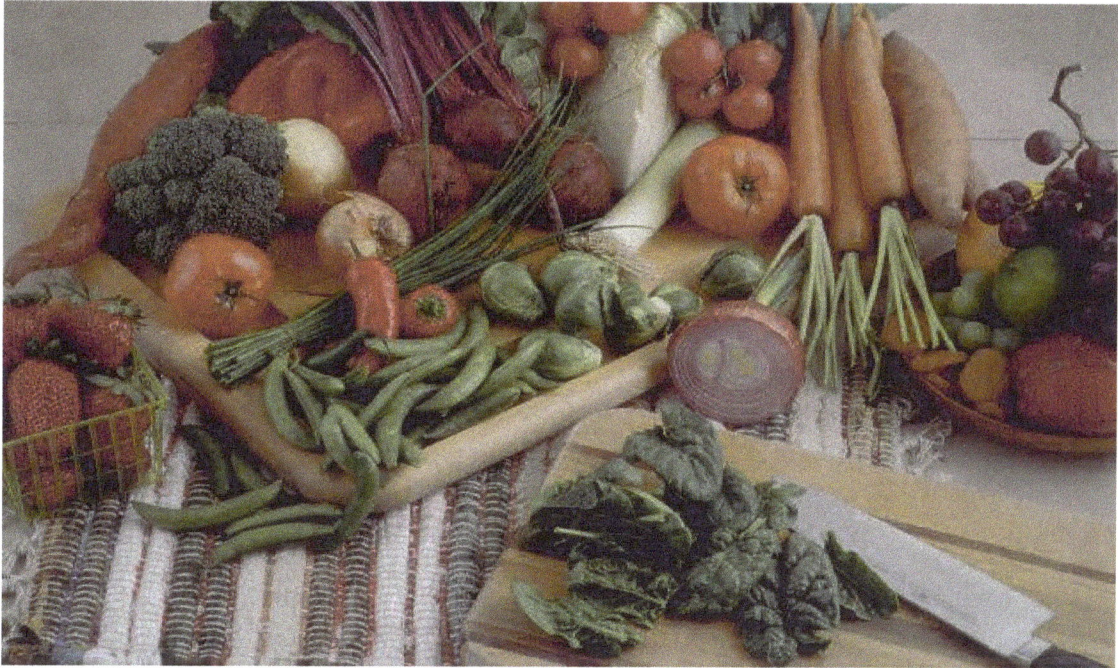

Food and Diet

Fundamentally, the best foods for physical nourishment and health are living, whole foods as they are provided by nature.

In the Hierarchy of Nutrients, foods and diet comprise food groups 2, 3, 4, and 5. To refresh your memory, Nutrient Group 2 contains natural raw foods, Nutrient Group 3 contains grains and legumes, Nutrient Group 4 contains flesh foods and dairy products, and Nutrient Group 5 contains refined and processed foods.

Fundamentally, the best foods for physical nourishment and health are living, whole foods as they are provided by nature. All the knowledge we have gained since the beginning of time continually supports this simple fact. Nature, in the form of plant foods, supplies all the food and medicine we need for physical health. Nature provides the most perfect food laboratory that yields an abundant menu of wholesome vitamins, minerals, proteins, carbohydrates, fats and other essential known and unknown nutrients. Fruits, vegetables, nuts, grains, seeds, and edible herbs, properly prepared and in adequate amounts, supply all the nutrients required for developing and maintaining optimum health.

What are the Best Foods to Eat?

Following is a list of dietary guidelines to help you choose the best nourishment for your body.

Plant Foods are the Best Nutrient Sources

Plant food nutrients have the right balance for your body, provided the soil is healthy. Plant foods contain all the necessary vitamins, minerals, proteins, carbohydrates, fats, and other known and unknown nutrients. They are balanced by nature for best compatibility with human ingestion, digestion, metabolism, assimilation, and elimination. Plant foods are low in calories, low in fat, low in sodium, high in potassium, high in antioxidants, and high in fiber, other important minerals, cofactors, and nutrients.

Raw Foods are Better Than Cooked Foods

Raw foods provide the highest nutrient value when eaten fresh. They should be from an organically rich soil free from harmful insecticides and contaminants. A high amount of raw food in our daily diet is essential to optimum health. The more we learn, the more our knowledge is reinforced that nature is the most superior food manufacturer. All the essential nutrients for the optimum health of humans are sun-cooked into the foods in Nature's kitchen.

Whole Foods are Superior to Processed and Refined Foods

For practical purposes, some cooked foods are an important part of the diet, especially in temperate and cold climates. In this case, whole foods, prepared most simply and naturally, are the best complement to a primarily raw food diet. However, all processed, refined, overcooked, over-manipulated and poorly combined foods should be excluded from the diet because they compromise health. They are deficient in essential nutrients, offer poorly balanced nutrients and/or add additional waste for your body to manage.

Popular processed foods like pasteurized milk, cheese, meat-substitute vegetarian foods, sugary breakfast cereals and canned foods are all inferior to whole, unprocessed food prepared simply and naturally. Scientifically manufactured or processed fruits, vegetables, grains, and juices are also compromised in nutrient value. But frozen whole, natural foods come close to being very similar to fresh foods. A good principle to follow is that whole foods build whole bodies. Processed and refined foods erode health, and build "unwhole" bodies.

Variety of Foods

For optimum health, we should choose a large variety of whole foods from Nature's menu. Variety ensures a greater spectrum of valuable nutrients that provide balance and more complete nutritional support, and makes a diet interesting. Vitamins and minerals in most foods are examples of nutrients that can have harmful effects on the body if they are provided in isolated forms. A more dramatic example is herbs which have therapeutically active ingredients (the basis of most pharmaceuticals). When isolated, these ingredients may be toxic if not carefully managed. Whole food variety is an effective strategy against excessive buildup of waste and unbalanced nutrients. This variety maximizes the spice, and minimizes the vice, in our diets.

Avoid Unnatural and Non-foods

All re-engineered foods, processed, and refined foods are unnatural. They drain your body's life force by making your body work harder to eliminate them, and compromise the processes for maintaining a healthy, disease-free body. Some of the more common items belonging to this list include all mechanically- and chemically-produced foods, sugar, caffeinated beverages, alcoholic beverages, and synthetic vitamins and minerals (especially, over-the-counter coal tar derivatives).

Many of the items in the above list may seem surprising and controversial at first glance due to the large amount of misleading information available. However, close examination and further study will reveal that they compromise the principle that only natural, whole plant foods, in the proper balance, and adequate amounts, provide the best nutrients for long-term health and wellness. Good scientific study and history prove this point.

There Are No "Magic" or "Health" Foods

There is no such thing as a magic food or health food. Food is simply a raw material used by the body for supporting a variety of metabolic, healing and rebuilding functions. Food in and of itself has no magical power and must be considered in the perspective of overall lifestyle factors. Given natural foods and the proper nutritional environment, your body has the ability to heal itself.

The key point is that there is no magic vitamin, mineral, herbal or other food therapy that causes health. However, several vital foods contain a broad spectrum of nutrients that provide excellent support and fill in the gaps of an otherwise well-balanced, whole-food diet. These vital foods include bee pollen, royal jelly, chlorella, wheat grass, and many edible herbs that have excellent healing properties. An optimally balanced whole-food diet consists primarily of fruits and vegetables with the addition of grains, nuts, seeds, and legumes to meet individual needs and capacities.

Juicing

Natural fruit and vegetable juices are both highly nutritious and beneficial, and when used as a meal can provide great digestive relief, nourishment, and therapeutic value. Juicing provides your body with a high concentration of nutrients in an easy-to-ingest form. Fresh fruit juices tend to support the cleansing ability of your body, and fresh vegetable juices tend to support the healing processes of your body. Fresh juices in proper combinations have an alkalizing effect on your body. The slightly alkaline state promotes optimum health of your body. There are a number of excellent books with recipes for refreshing, healthy, and therapeutic juice combinations. Some of these can be found in the back of this book.

The Ideal Diet

Obviously, there is no such thing as the ideal diet that works perfectly for everyone. Just as we all have unique talents and characteristics, we all have unique nutritional requirements. However, general characteristics can be applied to all of us. Key factors to be considered in formulating the ideal diet are:

- Your state of health
- Your lifestyle and environment
- Your desired health goals

Once these factors are determined, the common characteristics of the ideal diet can be structured to meet specific requirements. The ideal diet does not require weighing and measuring since it focuses more on individual needs, as opposed to, satiating an unnatural appetite. However, if the ideal diet were to be measured, it would tend to have the following profile. It would be

- High in water content and complex carbohydrates (over 80 percent)
- Low in fat (5–10 percent)
- Low in protein (5–10 percent)
- Comprised of as much raw food as possible, based on practicality, availability, season, and individual requirements.

Fruits and vegetables, grains, legumes, nuts and seeds, prepared in a simple and natural manner, are the best sources for the ideal diet. Individuals who are more sedentary or mentally active will benefit from a predominantly fruit and vegetable-based diet. At the same time, elite athletes could do well on a more complex diet, consisting of more grains, fats, and proteins. Infants and pregnant women may also need a little more protein in their diets. Protein and fat requirements are significantly less than most published guidelines and should be carefully evaluated before including them at higher than 5 percent of a whole food natural diet. A well-balanced vegetarian diet of sufficient calories provides more than adequate essential protein and fat requirements.

There are a number of ways to evaluate the ideal diet for different lifestyles. Mother's milk is probably the best model for demonstrating nutrient requirements. It is high in natural water (87 percent by volume), with the remaining 13 percent comprised of complex carbohydrates (sugar), fats, protein, vitamins, and minerals. The approximate non-water nutrient breakdown is as follows:

- 7 percent carbohydrates
- 3.5 percent fat
- 1.5 percent protein
- 1 percent vitamins and minerals.

Mother's milk is higher in complex carbohydrates and lower in concentrated fat and protein than cow's milk. The vitamin and mineral levels are relatively low, but completely sufficient and optimally balanced for growth during the fastest and most important development of the newborn baby. Fruits, and then vegetables, have the most comparable profile to mother's milk, making them the most important part of the ideal diet.

Fruits tend to support the cleansing functions of your body with their relatively higher sugar-water content. Vegetables tend to support the rebuilding processes of your body with their generally higher mineral water content. Your ideal diet should contain a rich supply of these health-supporting foods to meet your unique requirements.

The amount of fat and protein is considerably less in the ideal diet than in the Standard American Diet—less than 6 percent of the total food volume of mother's milk compared to over 60 percent of the Standard American Diet. Fat and protein are both important, but they are generally much overused, as in the typical fast food-oriented approach to eating. Though better than the Standard American Diet, the U.S. dietary guidelines are still too rich and stressful for the body. The ideal diet provides the best opportunity for optimum health. The following table shows a comparison of the Standard American Diet to the U.S. Dietary Guidelines and The Ideal Diet.

Comparison: Standard American Diet, U.S. Dietary Guidelines, and the Ideal Diet

The Standard American Diet allows almost anything edible (material that never existed until the last few decades – preservatives, additives, refined and artificial sugars, processed foods, etc.) to be eaten, and this results in a host of conditions and diseases. These problems include various cancers, strokes, high blood pressure, coronary artery disease, asthma, allergies, obesity, cardiovascular diseases, adult-onset diabetes mellitus, osteoporosis, arthritis, gallbladder disease, gout, Alzheimer's disease, leaching of calcium and other important minerals, and other degenerative conditions.

Table 1. Diet Type Comparisons

	Standard American Diet	U.S. Dietary Guidelines*	Ideal Diet
Protein(Source)	High (70–150+ g) 70% animal	High (70–100 g) (Not included)	Low (15–35 g)100% plant
Fat (% calories)**	High (35–45%)	Lower (< 30%)	Low (<10%)
Cholesterol	High (600–1000 mg/d)	Lower(< 300 mg/d)	None
Refined Sugar	High	Lower	None
Fiber	Low (10–15 mg)	Up to 25–30 mg	High (40–80 mg)
Food Sources	Mostly animal sources. Highly processed and much cooking with fats	Fewer animal sources. Processed More plant sources	All plant sources. Minimal or no processing
Calories	2,000–3,000+/day	Approximately the same	Calories based on lifestyle factors

*Mostly from U.S. Dietary Guidelines but supplemented with similar recommendations from other U.S. government sources

** Saturated fats, mostly from animal sources, are high in the Western diet. The U.S. Dietary Guidelines recommend a better balance of mono and polyunsaturated fats, which are more common in plant sources. The Ideal Diet achieves balance naturally.

The U.S. Dietary Guidelines recommend a modest restriction on saturated fats, high cholesterol foods, seasonings, and stimulants, which results in fewer degenerative conditions and diseases.

The Ideal Diet recommends fruits, vegetables, grains, legumes, nuts, seeds, and edible herbs, in proper combinations to meet individual needs and capacities, resulting in optimum health with the fewest degenerative conditions. This diet, properly combined, simply prepared, and derived from healthy soil, contains all the vitamins, minerals, complex carbohydrates, essential fatty acids, and essential amino acids required for total physical health.

Processed foods, white sugar, white flour, and all refined foods are extremely stressful to your body. They are both deficient in essential nutrients and add significant waste that must be eliminated for the attainment of optimum health. White sugar is particularly harmful and contributes to a host of physical and mental conditions.

The following table contains examples of the types of foods found in the standard American diet compared to the ideal diet.

Table 2. Comparison: Standard American Diet and The Ideal Diet

	Standard American Diet	Ideal Diet
Fruit	Sweetened fruit juice, carbonated drinks, canned fruit with syrup, desserts	Whole fruits - melons, kiwis, pineapples, oranges, apples, peaches, pears, plums, grapes, cherries, bananas, figs, dates
Vegetables	Potato chips, fried potatoes; canned corn, peas, and other vegetables; meat substitutes; canned vegetable juices, soups	Fresh broccoli, potatoes, carrots, celery, lettuce, squash, cucumbers, peppers, parsley, okra, string beans; fresh juices, soups
Grains	Refined cereal, white rice, white bread, pasta, white flour products, refined honey, alcoholic beverages	Oatmeal, brown rice, corn, amaranth, millet, grain bread, barley, rye, buckwheat, other whole grains
Protein	Beef steak, pork chops, bacon, chicken, fish, cold cuts, sausages, pastrami, hot dogs, hamburgers	Beans - soy, pinto, lentil, lima, green, red, black, adzuki
Dairy, Eggs	Cow's milk - whole, low-fat and skim; cheese, sour cream, cottage cheese, eggs, ice cream, yogurt, salad dressings	Homemade milk substitutes - rice, soy, almond, cashew; vitari (fruit "ice cream"); nut creams, sauces
Fats, sugars	Butter, margarine, candy bars, cookies, cake, pies, jelly, BBQ sauces, doughnuts, desserts, snack foods	Olives, avocados, olive oil, grain butter (e.g., millet); dried fruit - figs, dates, apricots; nuts, nut butters
Other	Coffee, tea, soda, alcohol, most fruit and "energy" drinks	Water, herb teas, coffee substitutes, natural fruit juices

The Ideal Diet: Nature's Hierarchical Model

The best rule is to use nature as our model for the ideal diet. We live on planet Earth and nature provides all our essential nutrients very efficiently and effectively. Based on this principle, the most abundantly available nutrients, provided by nature in order of availability and ease of consumption, are:

- Air
- Water
- Sunlight
- Earth's magnetic field
- Fruits
- Vegetables
- Nuts and seeds
- Grains
- Legumes (beans and peas)
- Flesh foods
- Dairy products

As described earlier, the above nutrients or food sources can be broken into four food groups. As noted, the first category includes the first four nutrients. They are so abundant and available that we generally take them for granted without realizing their significance in helping us experience high vitality and health.

Natural raw foods—fruits, vegetables, nuts, and seeds—are the second category of essential foods that are provided abundantly in an easy-to-consume form.

The third category—grains and legumes—generally requires some form of preparation for consumption. Their value, however, is that they contain highly concentrated nutrients (primarily complex carbohydrates and proteins) and can be stored for long periods of time in the event of flood, famine, or other factors affecting the availability of nature's primary foods. When practical, the highest nutrient value is provided by sprouting this category of foods, since cooking them will usually compromise their nutrient integrity.

The fourth, and last, category of nature's provision contains meat and dairy foods. These foods provide the most concentrated nutrients (primarily fats and proteins) and cause stress to our bodies. They should be eaten in very limited quantities, if at all. They are not essential for optimum health.

Refined and processed products are not provided by nature. They are really junk foods in a category by themselves and are the most compromising to human health.

As discussed earlier, the most nutritious food provided by nature for the initial nurturing of the human species is mother's milk. It provides all the nourishment needed for the optimum growth and vitality of the newborn infant. Mother's milk is primarily a high-water content food that includes all the essential nutrients, in the proper balance, and in an easy-to-consume form. It requires no preparation and is available in adequate amounts from healthy mothers for the first five years of an infant's life.

Fruits, vegetables, nuts, and seeds are the closest in nutrient composition to mother's milk. As you progress through the Hierarchy of Nutrients of natural or earth foods to other types of foods, you depart further from the nutrient content and composition of mother's milk. The category of processed foods consists of "food" not produced by our planet. Processed foods differ considerably in nutrient content and composition and are the most compromising to achieving and maintaining optimum health.

The Ideal Diet and Ideal Body Weight

Following the ideal diet, one will probably reach an ideal body weight. This is because the ideal diet can be used both as a reducing and a building diet. The appropriate combinations of food from plant sources, in the proper quantities, with an appropriate exercise program will reduce weight for the overweight and build healthy weight for the underweight. Over a period of time, the ideal diet will result in adjusting your body to its ideal weight.

A natural plant-based diet balances the metabolic processes in such a way that the body seeks the optimum weight to match your lifestyle. With strenuous physical activity like weightlifting or other labor-intensive work, a plant-based diet of adequate calories will produce a strong, muscular body. On the other hand, with a more sedentary lifestyle and modest exercise, an adequate plant-based diet will produce an optimum and healthy body weight.

Unfortunately, the whole topic of diet plays too large a role in our society. There are a number of formulas, including height/weight tables and body typing which are used to determine ideal weight ranges. The best approach would be to forget the height/weight tables and formulas and pursue the ideal diet components and combinations that yield the best physical, mental, and spiritual performance. With appropriate food choices, you can eat as much as you like without feeling starved or stuffed. This will reduce the stress of having to measure calories and chase after physically and mentally exhausting diet regimens. In addition, it will yield good health and your ideal weight.

The Ideal Diet and Carbohydrate Requirements

Unlike fats and proteins, there are no published guidelines for carbohydrate requirements. Our body's highest requirement and most efficient fuel are found in carbohydrate foods. Your carbohydrate requirements are based on a variety of factors, including level of health and activity. A diet consisting primarily of fruits and vegetables provides the best source of carbohydrates to support the nourishment and the waste elimination processes of your body.

The Ideal Diet and Protein Requirements

The amount of protein required after development is significantly lower than what it takes for initial development. The protein requirement for humans is highest in infancy when we experience our fastest growth. The dairy and meat industries, and misinformed health professionals, have been very successful in leading us to believe that our protein requirements are much higher than they are. Mother's milk is approximately 2.37% protein for the first six months of breastfeeding and drops to 1.07% after six months. This is a clear demonstration of nature's response to protein requirements in the fastest growing period of our lives.

Our protein requirements are as little as 10–25 grams per day, whereas the Standard American Diet may be as high as 100–200 grams per day. Excess protein leads to kidney problems, high blood levels of uric acid, ammonia, and other harmful acids, dehydration, and compromised immune system function. Calcium and other trace elements neutralize the excess acid that can lead to osteoporosis, arthritis, and other bone and joint degenerative processes. On the other hand, our protein requirements can be completely satisfied by a vegetarian-based diet of sufficient calories.

The Ideal Diet and Fat Requirements

Our bodies require very little dietary fat. Small amounts are required for the storage of fat-soluble vitamins and proper cholesterol and hormone balance. Our actual requirement for fat intake is less than 5 percent. The standard American diet contains 35–45 percent fat, most of which is derived from saturated animal sources and is high in cholesterol. Most fruits and vegetables are 1–5 percent fat, low in saturation, with virtually no cholesterol. If you include a small avocado and/or 1–2 ounces of nuts/seeds or olives every day (though these are not necessary every day) to meet your dietary fat requirements, your fat intake will be as much as 10–25 percent. This fat, however, is high-quality fat that is in harmony with the digestive system.

The worst kinds of fats in the diet are saturated (found only in meat and dairy products), trans fats, and partially hydrogenated fats. Many junk foods use partially hydrogenated fats as a preservative. The use of these fats leads to a host of degenerative disease processes, including cardiovascular conditions, high blood pressure, diabetes mellitus, and obesity.

The Ideal Diet as Medicine

The ideal diet provides both food and medicine for your optimum health. Drugs tend to suppress the immune system and are stressful to your body. In some instances, however, pharmaceuticals are the best strategy to pursue, especially for certain acute and painful conditions. If you experience any dramatic or persistent symptoms that might indicate infection or malfunction of a vital organ, it is important to see a qualified physician for a complete physical exam, tests, and appropriate medicine.

However, drugs are generally used excessively and inappropriately. Special care in understanding the health implications of drugs, vaccinations, inoculations, elective surgery, X-rays, and related approaches is necessary for promoting and sustaining optimum health. In all instances, the Physicians' Desk Reference (PDR), a drug reference that your doctor and the library have, should be consulted to find out about a drug's specific uses and side effects.

Let food be your medicine. Most lifestyle problems respond best to proper diet, gentle natura therapy, and lifestyle modification. In proper amounts and combinations, plant sources contain all the food and medicine required for total health. There are many herbs and homeopathic remedies that, when taken properly, are a much safer and more effective medicine, especially when combined with other dietary and lifestyle factors. The ideal diet supports your body's healing processes. Drugs, medicine protocols, isolated vitamin and mineral therapies, and surgery should be used as last resorts where simpler measures may not be appropriate.

The Ideal Diet and Vitamin, Mineral, and Herbal Supplements

The ideal diet, in the proper combinations and with sufficient variety, contains all the vitamins, minerals, and other essential nutrients required for optimum performance and health. There is no biochemist in the world who can figure out with precision the accuracy and balance of essential nutrients required by your body better than nature.

Care should be exercised always when taking supplements, especially synthetic, fractionated supplements. Most synthetic vitamin and mineral supplements can be harmful when taken in an isolated form apart from whole foods. Intemperate and indiscriminate use of supplemental products can lead to both imbalances and toxicity. When properly included, high-quality vitamin and mineral supplement products made from reputable sources using quality processing techniques can be excellent additions to, but not substitutes for, a healthy and holistic diet and lifestyle. A healthy body will actually create many of the needed known and unknown nutrients through balanced, interactive, and adaptive metabolic processes.

Evaluating Criteria for Dietary Supplements

The following are the key criteria for evaluating the integrity and effectiveness of supplements from a natural health perspective:

- It should be produced by nature. Nature is the best intermediary for all nutrients that affect optimum human performance. Biochemistry and food technologists can never improve on the superior power of nature's harmonizing and bioavailable formulations.

- It should be produced in the most natural setting. Clean air, water, appropriate sunlight, and a micronutrient-rich soil, uncompromised by pesticides and other harmful intrusions, are key. All contribute to the integrity and effectiveness of a dietary supplement.

- It should be harvested at the right time. This ensures that it is mature and complete, as nature intended for optimum bioavailability of active ingredients.

- It should be taken in its most natural form. Processing should be minimized, ensuring that no unnatural substances, preservatives, or other "enhancers" are added, while maintaining the integrity of its active ingredients.

- It should be from a reliable source. Check with your naturopathic doctor for reliable supplement companies.

- If possible, the packaging should be environmentally friendly.

Summary Remarks on Whole Food Supplements

As a naturopath, I am uncompromising in the principle that optimum health requires balanced observance of the natural essentials of health. Among those essentials are clean air, water, sunlight, magnetic energy, proper nutrition, exercise, rest, mental, emotional and spiritual factors – all in moderation. Unfortunately, we experience different levels of compromise in all these areas and, consequently, experience compromises to our health and well-being. These compromised conditions range from tolerable to severe and, for many, affect their quality of life. While dietary and lifestyle factors are the most effective of all health modalities, it is clear that the right kind of supplementation can assist many people in helping them address the consequences of dietary and lifestyle indiscretions.

There are several high-nutrient foods, vitamins, minerals, and herbs available that can offer nutritional support for compromised diets or health conditions. Some of the popular ones are bee pollen, noni juice, goji juice, mangosteen juice, wheat grass juice, echinacea, goldenseal, ginseng, other selected herbs (including their teas, tinctures and extracts), and many more. Whole food supplements are the best strategy for deficiency and compromised health conditions. These products can be effective when incorporated with a strategy that employs many principles outlined here.

A Word on Meat and Dairy Products

There is much misinformation and many misconceptions about the role of meat and dairy products in the diet. The meat and dairy industries are very large and powerful, and play a significant role in our dietary practices. The following are some important factors regarding these products:

Problems with Meat Products

All flesh foods (which include beef, poultry, fish, pork, etc.) are different from fruits and vegetables with regard to their nutrient content and balance. For example, flesh foods are high in calories, high in fat, high in the wrong kind of protein, high in sodium, and low in potassium. Fruits and vegetables are low in calories, low in fat, adequate in essential protein, low in sodium, and high in potassium. Your body is designed to function best on the latter formula.

All flesh foods are in some state of decomposition and lower in nutrient value (usually overcooked) when compared to natural plant-based foods. They also place a significant waste burden on the system due to the large amounts of hormones, antibiotics, and feed pesticides used in modern meat production.

Even though all flesh foods have more concentrated proteins than plant-based foods, they are not optimally balanced and place a harmful burden on the digestive system. If consumed at all, flesh foods should be treated as a condiment and not a main meal. All the amino acids needed by your body are adequately provided in plant foods eaten in adequate amounts.

Problems with Dairy Products

Cow's milk, especially pasteurized and homogenized, is poorly balanced for optimum digestion and utilization. Mother's milk is optimally balanced in protein, fat, calcium, potassium, phosphorus, and other important nutrients for nurturing infants. Certain fruit and vegetable juices are better sources of nutrients than cow's milk where mother's milk is an impractical choice.

Pasteurized milk is deficient in important enzymes required for its proper digestion and bioavailability of its nutrients. It is highly mucus-forming and acidic. Like whole milk, pasteurized milk curdles and becomes solid as soon as it enters the stomach. In addition, it combines poorly with most foods. Pasteurization does reduce the risk of certain fatal diseases, but the important question is, "Why would you want to nourish yourself with the food of a diseased animal or its output?"

Homogenization pulverizes milk components, allowing easier absorption of harmful substances and resulting in high cholesterol, respiratory, vascular, and other conditions.

The labeling of "low-fat" milk misleads the general public. The dairy industry uses a different standard of measurement than the rest of the food industry. Dairies measure by volume weight including water content rather than the fat content of total calories. Effectively, whole milk (which is 3.3 percent fat by volume) is actually 49 percent fat as to percentage of calories; low-fat 2-percent milk is actually 35 percent fat. Only non-fat or skim milk is actually lower than 5 percent fat. However, by taking out the fat, milk is altered from a high-fat to a high-protein food. Milk protein is very stressful to human digestion and may be even more harmful than the fat content of milk. The following table shows the fat, protein, and carbohydrate contents of whole, low-fat, and skim milk as a percentage of calories. Mother's milk, which is the ideal food for nursing infants, is also included for comparison to cow's milk.

Table 3. Comparison: Milk Types

	Whole	Low-Fat (2%)	Low-Fat (1%)	Skim	Mother's Milk
Fat	49%	35%	23%	4%	28%
Protein	21%	26%	31%	39%	15%
Carbohydrates	30%	39%	46%	57%	57%

Mother's milk is higher in carbohydrates and lower in fat and protein than whole cow's milk. Skim milk is considerably lower in fat, but also much higher in protein than mother's milk. After the first six months of breastfeeding, the fat and protein content of the mother's milk decreases while the carbohydrate percentage increases. This may be nature's way of telling us that our fat and protein requirements, while modest to begin with, are the highest during the early months of breastfeeding. Processed dairy products are even higher in fat and/or protein concentration than cow's milk since much of the water is eliminated during processing.

The nutrient value of all dairy products is derived from the plant foods the animal has eaten. Today, harmful non-food substances, such as pesticides, antibiotics, and growth hormones, usually compromise the commercial cow's diet of mostly plant-based food, and are then passed on to us. Therefore, cow's milk contains nutrients in an incorrect balance and is also likely to contain harmful substances, thus leading to compromised health.

Dairy products can be extremely stressful to the body, and, for some people, they cause abnormally fast and/or excessive growth. This growth, however, is often at the expense of long-term vitality and health. If consumed at all, dairy products should be taken in very small quantities, sourced from healthy cows, and in its whole, unprocessed, and raw form.

Meat and Dairy Requirements for Athletes

Many athletes are under the misconception that flesh and dairy products are required for strength, energy, stamina, and overall athletic performance. Many studies and the successes of several world-class vegetarian athletes demonstrate this long-held misconception's fallacy. One example is Andreas Cahling, the Swedish bodybuilder who won both the Mr. Europe and Mr. Universe titles. He was a pure frugivore. He ate fruit before, during, and after his training. He ate no meat or dairy products, and not even grains or vegetables. In this context, it is important to understand that several foods are mistakenly categorized as vegetables that botanically are fruits. Cucumbers, avocados, tomatoes, squash and all seed-bearing plants are correctly classified as fruits, not vegetables.

I am not advocating a pure fruitarian diet for optimal athletic performance, since many fruits have been hybridized to match our appetite for sweets. It is important to consume fruits based on individual capacities. This will help you avoid stressful digestive, pancreatic, and adrenal conditions, including hypoglycemia. A good rule for high fruit consumption is to buffer the high sugar content with compatible vegetables such as lettuce, cucumbers and/or celery. See the appendix on food combining for more information on how to eat fruits properly. Nuts and seeds, as well as nut and seed milks, are also excellent additions to a predominantly fruit and vegetarian diet for optimal athletic performance.

In his book God's Way to Ultimate Health, Dr. George A. Malkmus lists several world- class athletes, all holders of world records in their fields, who all happen to be vegetarians. These include Dave Scott, six-time winner of the Ironman Triathlon (and the only man to win it twice); Sixto Linares, world record holder in the 24-hour marathon; Paavo Nurmi, holder of 20 world records and nine Olympic medals in distance running; Robert Sweetgall, the world's premier ultra-distance walker; Murny Rose, world record holder in the 400 and 1,500 meter freestyle; Estelle Gray and Cheryl Marek, world record holders in cross-country tandem cycling; Henry Aaron, all-time major league home run champion; Stan Price, world record holder in the bench press; Roy Hilligan, Mr. America bodybuilding champion; Ridgely Abele, holder of eight national championships in karate; and Dan Millman, world champion gymnast. This list may surprise the average American, based on what we have been taught to believe about protein and meat.

There are many additional factors regarding the meat and dairy issue, such as rampant disease, antibiotics, hormone injections, compromised animal diets, as well as ecological, ethical and moral considerations. The vegetarian diet promotes total health for you, your neighbors, and your planet. There are several good books available, some of which are listed at the end of this book, that provide excellent coverage of this important topic.

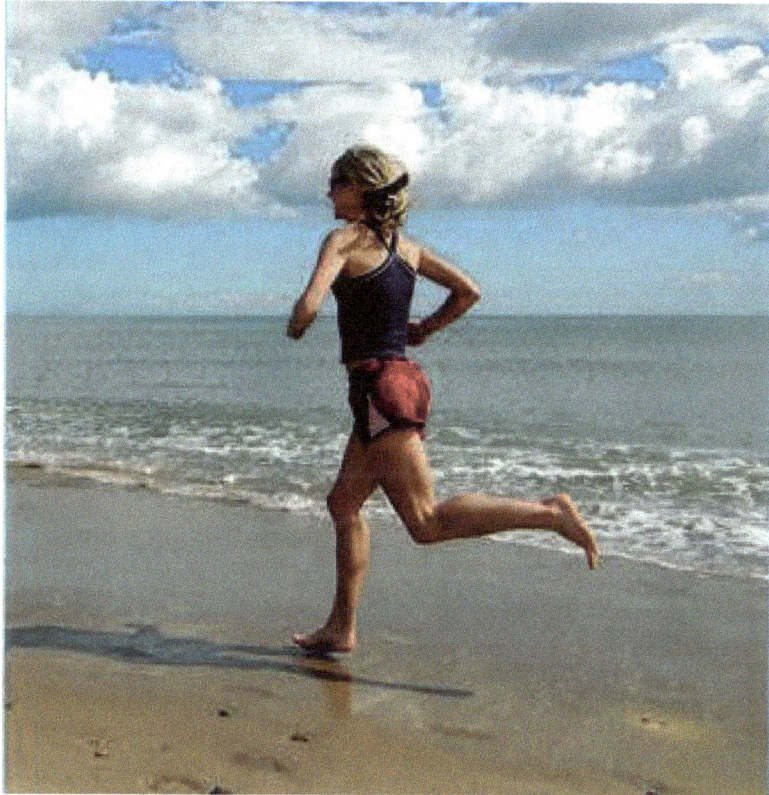

Exercise

Without movement, all life ceases to exist.

In addition to those things mentioned in the Nutrient Hierarchy, the body needs a proper amount of exercise and rest.

Exercise is another important support for the optimum performance of your body. It contributes to both nourishment of your body and the elimination of waste. The fundamental principle of exercise as it relates to health is movement. Without movement, all life ceases to exist. In death, all systems of your body – including the heart, brain, and circulatory systems – stop "moving." If anything in the universe stops moving, its function is altered. This underlying principle of movement is the factor that promotes and supports optimum health. Movement engages all the major systems in your body, including the muscular, skeletal, neural, glandular, and lymphatic systems.

From a nourishing point of view, exercise is often improperly pursued. For exercise to have positive health benefits, it should be enjoyable and done in moderation. Attitude is very important! Studies indicate that exercise that is performed as drudgery yields marginal health benefits, at best, and can lead to degenerative disease processes.

It is important to understand the difference between health and fitness. Fitness is more closely aligned with cardiovascular performance, muscle tone, body symmetry, strength, and related characteristics. Health implies functional and structural integrity of internal and external organs and systems, and avoidance of disease processes.

Most people generally use approximately 50 of the more than 600 muscles in their bodies. This often results in overuse of less than 10 percent of our muscles, and this can result in several disease processes. Using a variety of individualized exercises or movements (based on genetic or environmental conditions) offers many advantages to optimizing health and wellness.

Anything that encourages the natural movement of your body contributes to your health. The type and amount of exercise are subject to the same rules of temperance and balance as the foods we eat. Whether walking, running, swimming, weightlifting; gardening, or doing aerobics, yoga, tai chi, martial arts, or pursuing any other activity, the following principles contribute to a healthy approach to exercise. It should:

- Be enjoyable and relaxing
- Be free of strain and pain
- Use as many muscles and joints as is feasible
- Use a variety of movements
- Balance strength with flexibility and stretching
- Cause you to breathe deeply
- Ensure adequate rest.

Benefits of Exercise

Regular exercise is not only a preventive measure; it also helps us maintain health at its best. There are many benefits of physical exercise, which include the following:

- Exercise makes one more energetic and gives a sense of well-being.
- Exercise helps to lower high blood pressure. The New England Journal of Medicine published a study that found that aerobic exercise significantly lowered blood pressure in hypertensive patients.

- Exercise strengthens bones. Research on additive effects of weight-bearing exercise and estrogen on bone mineral density in older women was conducted at the Washington University School of Medicine in St. Louis, Missouri. The results of the study demonstrated that a woman can increase her bone mass by 2–3 percent per year by doing weight-bearing exercise.[1]

- Exercise promotes an increase in HDL (good) cholesterol. A study[2] of nearly 3,000 healthy, middle-aged men running a certain number of miles per week revealed that exercise was associated with higher HDL levels.

- Exercise helps in the management of diabetes. Harvard researchers documented that exercise decreases the risk of developing diabetes in adulthood. Exercise increases the ability of muscle membranes to transport glucose into muscle cells. This particular transportation is not dependent on insulin, thus lowering the insulin requirement.

- Exercise improves communication in those with Alzheimer's disease. In a study examining the communication skills of two groups of Alzheimer's patients, more than 40 percent of the group in a walking exercise program experienced significant improvement in communication skills; whereas the group who were given conversation lessons experienced no significant improvement.[3]

- Exercise improves mental health according to two studies.[4] Patients not suffering from Alzheimer's disease showed measurable improvement in memory in an aerobic exercise program of 9–10 weeks duration. With increased activity, older Americans showed improved mental function. There is a clear, linear relationship between the level of activity and the level of mental ability. Through regular, active use of the body, one can discover a greater sense of well-being, far greater vitality, and a calmer, more relaxed attitude toward daily pressures.

- Exercise improves cardiac function. It strengthens the heart, making it more efficient, pumping a greater volume of blood in each contraction.

- Exercise improves quality of life. A consensus panel convened by the National Institutes of Health identified other important benefits in quality of life from exercise such as better mental health, less stress, less anxiety and depression, and a decreased risk of certain cancers.

---

1   Kohrt WM, Snead DB, et al. Additive effects of weight-bearing exercise and estrogen on bone mineral density in older women,@ *J Bone Miner Res* 1995 Sep;10(9):1303-1311.

2   Kokkinos PF, Holland JC, et al. Miles run per week and high-density lipoprotein cholesterol levels in healthy, middle-aged men: a dose-response relationship,@ *Arch Intern Med* 1995 Feb 27;155(2):415- 420.

3   Friedman R, Tappen RM. The effect of planned walking on communication in Alzheimer's disease,@ J *Am Geriatr Soc* 1991 Jul;39(7):650-654.

4   Bowers RW, et. al. Memory Dependent Reaction Time and Improved Cardiovascular Fitness in Middle-Aged Adults.@ *Med Sci Sports Exerc* 1983;15:117.
Clarkson-Smith L, Hartley AA, Relationships between physical exercise and cognitive abilities in older adults,@ *Psychol Aging* 1989 Jun;4(2):183-189.

In 1998, *The Oregonian* published a story about an old man, Ben Levinson, 103 years old, who set a world record for the shot-put for men over 100. He threw the ball 10 feet and 1.25 inches. But for Ben the achievement was to be throwing at all, at over 100 years! Thirteen years before, Ben Levinson was a depressed, unfit 90-year-old, shuffling around, frail and obviously ready for the grave. Ben had become dependent and weak through lack of exercise. Fortunately for Ben, he met Dave Crawley, an athletics trainer, who challenged him to feel 80 again. Ben began a training program, walking 20 minutes a day at 2.5 miles per hour, and weight-training three or four times a week. He grew 2 inches, just with better posture and more confidence, says Crawley.

If a fitness program could do that for this 90-year-old, just think what it could do for you!

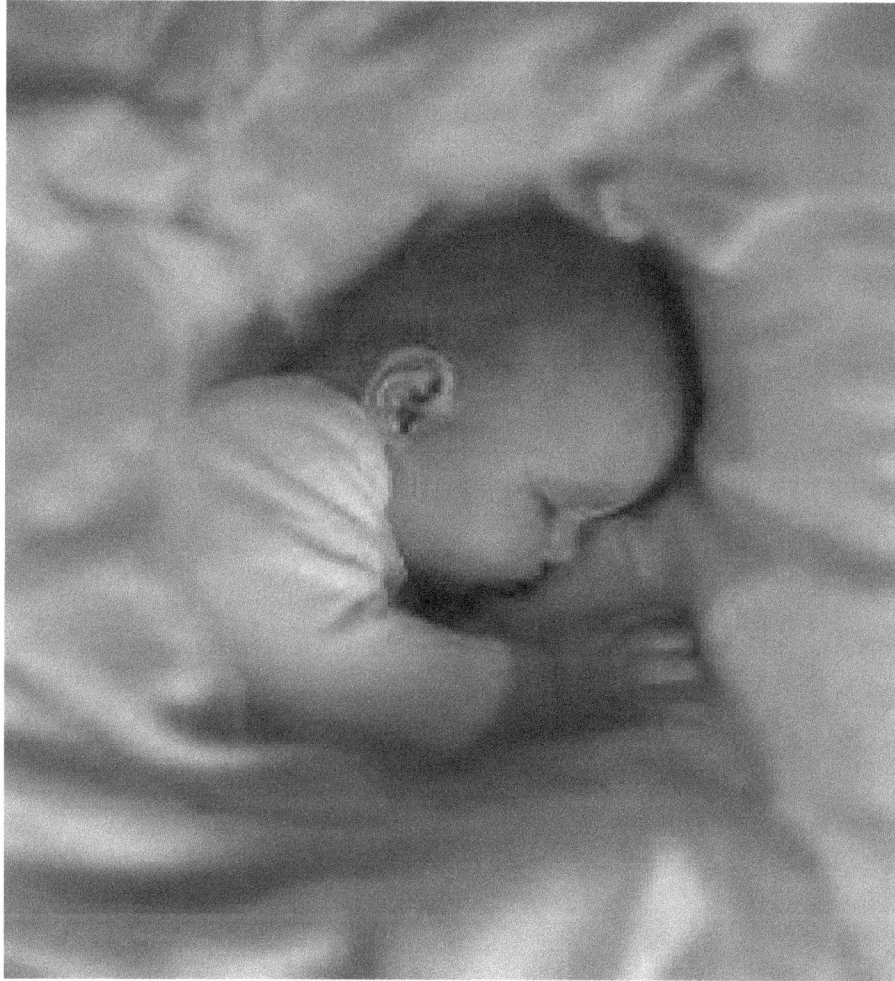

Rest

Relaxation techniques such as massage, meditation, and prayer provide valuable rest that contributes to our health.

Adequate rest is imperative for optimum health. Rest brings restoration and replenishes the resources we use. Without rest, the body's process of catabolism (breaking down) overrides that of anabolism (building up), resulting in disease and compromised health.

Sleep is the most important medium for rest. Short naps, peaceful and relaxing environments, and mental quietness all contribute to rest.

In one day, the average heart beats 110,000 times, and the blood runs through millions of miles of arteries, veins, and capillaries. We speak thousands of words, breathe 28,000 times, move major muscles hundreds of times, and operate some 15- 20 billion brain cells. No wonder sleep is important in restoring our energy and maintaining health. As Shakespeare wrote, "Sleep wraps up the raveled sleeve of care."

A newborn baby sleeps an average of 20 hours a day; a 6-year-old, 10 hours; a 12-year-old, 9 hours; and an adult, approximately 8 hours. Whether these averages are optimum varies, depending upon the individual. Breslow and Belloc in their famous Alameda County study, showed that persons obtaining 8–9 hours of sleep per night seemed to have better health outcomes than those sleeping for lesser or longer periods of time. Occasionally there are individuals, such as Ben Franklin and Thomas Edison, who can get by with 4 or 5 hours a night; these are the exceptions rather than the rule. Many who sleep these short periods of time at night take short catnaps throughout the day. Albert Einstein required at least 9 hours of sleep. Adequate sleep should remove sleepiness and drowsiness during the day and permit a sense of well-being and alertness.

Students who study all night prior to an examination often suffer the consequences of sleep deprivation manifested in inferior grades. Work schedules that do not permit adequate sleep may result in increased inattention in the workplace.

The area in the brainstem thought to cause sleep is the raphe nuclei in the lower half of the pons. Extensions proceed from these nuclei to most of the limbic system of the brain, the thalamus, as well as the hypothalamus and reticular system, and in their terminal ending the extensions release serotonin. Agents inhibiting serotonin formation are associated with an inability to sleep. Because of this finding, serotonin has been assumed to play a role in promoting sleep. Other neurotransmitters may play a role in sleep as well.

According to sleep experts, we go through various stages and certain cycles when we sleep. Each cycle lasts approximately 90 minutes. We start with stage-one sleep, the lightest stage, and then progress to a deeper, stage-two sleep. Stage-three sleep is related to delta wave brain activity, the slowest and most relaxed brain wave activity. Stage four is our deepest stage of sleep. The most powerful healing and rebuilding takes place during the fourth stage of sleep, which lasts approximately 20–45 minutes. Then, we gradually return through stage three, stage two, and stage one sleep. A complete and uninterrupted cycling through these stages allows us to awaken refreshed without an alarm clock, and significantly contributes to optimum health.

In cases of compromised health and excessive physical and mental activity, rest is imperative for restoring and supporting your body's natural healing ability. It is the most important activity or exercise for replenishing spent resources.

Hormones, in which secretion is influenced by sleep patterns include:

1. **Cortisol.** This hormone is secreted during sleep in the second half of the sleep period, in which it prepares the body for the activity of the next day. Cortisol has numerous effects, influencing blood glucose levels, regulating sodium and potassium concentrations, regulating blood pressure, and influencing muscle strength. Regular sleep habits result in regular patterns of cortisol secretion.
2. **Growth hormone.** This hormone is secreted at its maximal rate during sleep. There are effects of growth hormone on glucose and amino acid metabolism.
3. **Melatonin.** Secretion rates of this hormone increase during the night but may have more of a role to play in sexual regulation than anything to do with sleep regulation.

There are a number of factors that influence good sleep. These include:

- A quiet bedroom, free of bright light and noise, properly ventilated, and of a comfortable temperature, aids in sleeping.
- The time preceding retiring should be free of arguments, exciting TV, and stressful events. It should be a quiet time to wind down the day's activity.
- Regular exercise and the avoidance of excessive fatigue are helpful.
- The last meal of the day should be a light one and be taken a few hours prior to retiring.
- A warm, not hot, bath may help relaxation before going to bed.
- Avoidance of alcohol, tobacco, caffeine, and other chemical substances that interfere with the normal sleep patterns is advised.

A number of factors influence poor sleep, including:

- Irregularity in rising and going to bed, shift work, travel across time zones, and weekend sleep changes
- Medical conditions such as sleep apnea, respiratory disorders, cardiac conditions, phobias, and other psychiatric disorders, may require professional assistance.

The Bible recommends weekly rest, and such rest seems to provide a much-needed break from the tedium of work, as well as recognized productivity benefits. During World War II, increased productivity was achieved when the continuous, non-stop work schedule, to attempt increased production, was reduced to a 48-hour work week. The increase was about 15 percent and demonstrated that even under the pressures of war, people have limitations on their work capabilities.

On July 29, 1941, six months before the entry of the United States into the war, Prime Minister Winston Churchill announced in the House of Commons, "If we are to win this war it will be by staying power. For this reason we must have one holiday per week and one week holiday per year." And this was voted into law!

Periodic rests include annual vacations. These vacations are not necessarily periods of inactivity, but of engagement in activities normally outside the scope of the routine. These times provide mental and emotional restitution and help in creativity and family relationships.

There is a clear relationship between the Hierarchy of Nutrients and Rest. Adequate restful sleep requires good habits, such as eating properly, especially light suppers and avoiding stressful circumstances just before retiring. Supper should be eaten at least two hours (and as much as 3–4 hours) when eating complex and concentrated meals, before retiring. Dinner should be skipped or consist of something light, like fruit, if sufficient time is not available before retiring.

The digestive system tends to take up more energy than any other major system of your body, including the circulatory, respiratory, and nervous systems. Temperance in diet, proper food combining, and therapeutic fasting are some of the many energy-conserving and resting opportunities your body uses to repair and optimize the rest of its bodily functions and processes.

Use the many relaxation techniques, including massage, meditation, and prayer to provide valuable rest that contributes to health and wellness. In addition to natural sleep and a temperate diet and lifestyle, relaxation techniques contribute to vibrant energy and optimum health.

The Lord, our Creator, knows that our body needs balanced daily rest, physically, mentally, emotionally, and socially. He also knows that in order to function optimally we need weekly rest, as stated in Exodus 20:8-10: "Remember the Sabbath day, to keep it holy. Six days you shall labor and do all your work: but the seventh day is the Sabbath of the Lord your God: in it you shall do no work: you, nor your son, nor your daughter, nor your manservant, nor your maidservant, nor your cattle, nor your stranger who is within your gates."

The Lord wants us to have fellowship with Him, especially on the Sabbath day, for He has created us as His children. Part of the blessing of the Sabbath rest comes as we support and relate with each other. Service to others provides a powerful rest from the self-focused and egocentric activities that often encumber us. The Sabbath was made for man, not man for the Sabbath! Regular sleep and weekly rest empowers us to be receptive to the blessing of God so He can fill our lives with His many blessings!

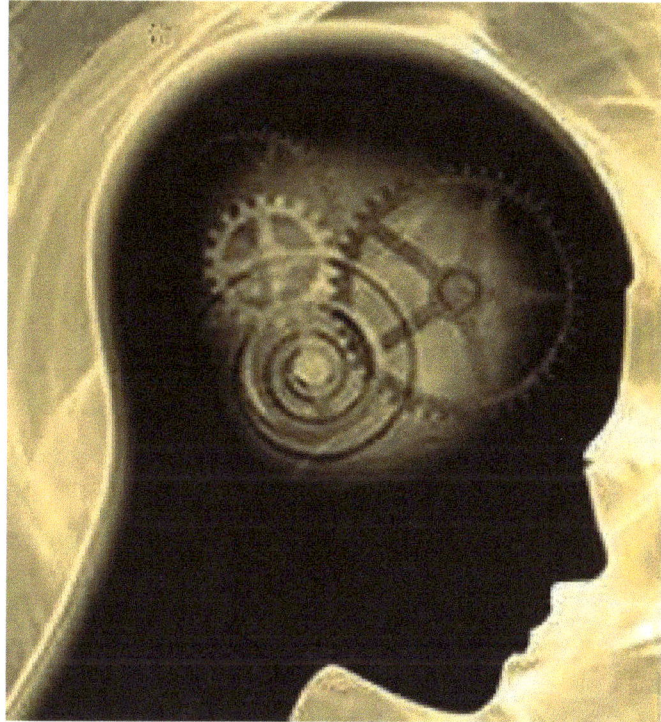

The Mind

Positive thinking and positive emotions have a profound effect on promoting and maintaining optimum health. The mind directs the operation of the autonomic nervous system, its neurotransmitters, the endocrine system, and its hormones for metabolic regulation. Neurotransmitters play an important role in emotions and behavior. Endorphins are neurotransmitters that are the body's natural pain relievers. The mind has many well-established and some unknown effects on the well-being of your body.

To quote a popular phrase, "the mind is a terrible thing to waste." There are many studies demonstrating the power of the mind. Positive thinking and positive emotions have a profound effect on promoting and maintaining optimum health. The mind directs the operation of the autonomic nervous system, its neurotransmitters, the endocrine system, and its hormones for metabolic regulation. Neurotransmitters play an important role in emotions and behavior.

Endorphins are neurotransmitters that are the body's natural pain relievers. The mind has many well-established and some unknown effects on the well-being of your body.

The mind can rule and modify bodily functions. We reflect what we think. A perfectly balanced mind can handle and detoxify a great burden. When you have a mind and nervous system free of anxiety, worry, and fear and are in a state of love, all cells within the system are in balance and harmony. Cells in harmony can eliminate and rebuild with great ease. Part of a mental purification program is to express, let go, feel joy, love without conditions, and forgive. This takes some effort for most of us, as there are many moods involved with changing wrongs that need to be righted and forgiving those who have done wrong things against us.

An open and accepting mind, supplemented with a sincere and humble heart, is the fast-track way of receiving this state of unconditional love. Unconditional and thorough love is found in the selfless seeking of the truth. This kind of love can free you of the mental stress that compromises your ability to achieve optimum health. It is very important to get your mind and heart in order to experience the highest level of vibrant health.

The power of the mind is considered in some health approaches, but has not been fully embraced by many conventional medical institutions and practitioners. The inseparable linkage of the mind to your body makes health at the mental level imperative for maintaining health at the physical level. The following are some aids for experiencing health at the mental level.

Positive Views of Self, Others, and the Environment

Looking to the positive, as in seeing the glass half full versus half empty, promotes health for you, your neighbor and your planet. Your perceptions and views shape the content and character of reality.

Positive Attitude Toward Health

Attitude shapes your experiences of health. Viewing yourself at different stages of health versus labeling yourself with diseases and related conditions is a healthier attitude.

Positive Emotions

Positive emotions nourish the body while negative emotions are harmful to your body. Love, joy, trust, hope, and forgiveness as opposed to anger, sadness, suspicion, despair, and revenge promote health and can reverse disease processes.

Visualization

Seeing yourself in the desired state of health generates the internal energetic and metabolic processes necessary for attaining the physical manifestations of your mental visualizations.

Support Groups

An environment that promotes a positive outlook can promote positive health benefits. Developing relationships that support your health philosophies and strategies enhances your realization of desired health goals.

Meditation

Calming and putting your mind at equilibrium and tranquility offers rest and opens your mind to higher achievements. A mind at rest engages the autonomic nervous system, specifically the parasympathetic system which encourages healing and improved metabolic function.

Prayer

Communication at the highest level of your being, with the Divine Power, promotes health beyond limited man-made remedies. This gives wholesome rest to your mind for the accomplishment of needed changes in your lifestyle. Prayer enhances and fortifies your life, taking health beyond physical and mental boundaries. It helps us to reach the highest levels of health and personal development.

The mind plays a pivotal role in the total health of the body. The mind is nourished by a pure and healthy body and through meditation and positive emotions. For optimum health at the mind level, our prayers and wishes must be harmonized with positive thoughts and actions.

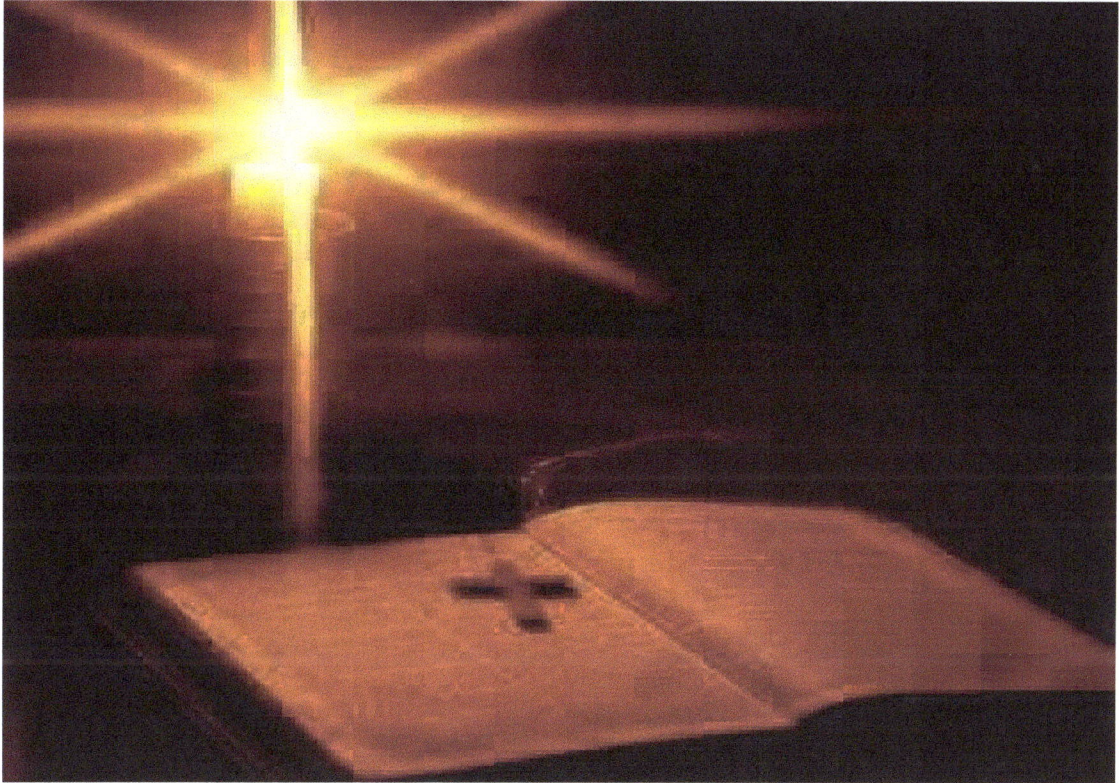

The Spirit

All great civilizations have been founded on religious beliefs and moral values leading to an orderly society. Belief in spiritual values is a strong motivator to treat others well and to develop peaceful human relationships. Studies indicate that those with regular spiritual practices who meet with a faith community live longer, live better, and are far less likely to have a stroke or heart attack. Faith can empower you to overcome stress and destructive habits. Trust and reliance in a loving powerful God give the ability to enjoy a healthful lifestyle. Complete belief in God permits Him to fill our lives with outrageous health!

Plant-based food nourishes your ***body***. A nourished body, in turn enriches the foundation for the growth of love and peace, which supports the optimum health of your ***mind***. Positive thoughts and emotions then help to nourish the environment for bearing the fruits of unconditional love, which supports the health of your ***spirit***.

All great civilizations have been founded on religious beliefs and moral values leading to an orderly society. Belief in spiritual values is a strong motivator to treat others well and to develop peaceful human relationships. History demonstrates thatfaithless and amoral societies become so corrupt that they cannot survive. Belief is characteristic of science as well as religion. Just as faith in a scientific principle is verified when tests show that its application leads to correct conclusions, so faith in God is validated when it brings satisfying results. Studies indicate that those with regular spiritual practices who meet with a faith community live longer, live better, and are far less likely to have a stroke or heart attack. Faith can empower you to overcome stress and destructive habits. Belief can give you peace of mind and enable you to reach your full potential through positive choices.

Everyone needs to believe in something lasting and stable for viability and long-term health. Health at the spiritual level synergistically produces health at all levels. Your mind is energized with the vibrant health of positive thinking and emotions. Your body is ruled by the mind, bent on fortifying sustenance versus subsistence, for the medium that gives it actuality.

There are many challenges we face at both the physical and mental levels that can compromise our ability to focus on our spiritual growth and development. Like air, which is abundantly supplied and easily available, the spirit element of our being is easy to take for granted and overlook, even though it has so pervasively and abundantly provided for our life and well-being.

Spiritual realization is available to all who are seeking wisdom and truth. Many will squander this powerful and abundantly provided path to total health, but the few who truly set aside some quiet time to embrace the perfect and mysterious aspect of the spirit, will find it. "Ask and it will be given to you, seek and you will find, knock at the door and it will be opened to you,"—Matthew 7:7-9. When you hear the prompting of your spirit with a pure mind and heart listen to it and abide by it, it will grow and reward you with renewed health and wellness.

The spiritual life force is available to all of us, regardless of station in life or level of performance. This aspect of our being puts us all on a level playing field. It is the most powerful force of our being. An ounce of spiritual health can transcend pounds of physical and mental protocols. Many mysterious and miraculous cures testify to this truly awesome phenomenon. Those who are wise enough to accept and capitalize on this aspect of our being can create the physiological and mental nutrients to overcome obstacles to achieving optimum health.

Spiritual growth and nourishment is a major aspect of many religions or philosophies. There are many paths that mankind has experienced during our quest for spiritual realization. Many sincere and well-intentioned religious organizations try to claim sole ownership of the spirit, just as certain health institutions try to own all aspects of our diet and health. This often leads to judgmental, condescending, political, and other compromising factors that are the waste material that must be eliminated for healthy spiritual growth and wellness. The wisdom of men and institutions will always fall short of the enormous wisdom and power of the Creator of men and their institutions.

Relying solely on human knowledge, science and its institutions will always compromise total health at all levels, especially the spiritual level.

The mysteries still to be unraveled far outweigh the knowledge we have gained during our brief history. Spiritual health that is pure, peaceful, loving, and sincere is available to each of us. While the spirit part of our being is the most powerful aspect of human existence, it tends to be both extremely complex and underutilized by many, and yet simple and powerfully utilized by some.

What causes us to fall short of capitalizing on our spiritual support and nourishment? Don't we all want total health and happiness in our lives? The questions are easy, but the answers are not as simple. There are many distractions, including the daily activities involved in feeding, sheltering, and providing for our livelihoods, our natural pleasure-seeking ways, and other factors affected by our neighbors and environment. At another level, our own pride, selfish motives, arrogant sense of self-worth and refusal to accept truth can also act as stressful burdens requiring elimination for true spiritual health.

Once we understand and appreciate our relative insignificance from a universal perspective and humbly submit to and accept the spiritual prompting of a pure and healthy mind, we engage in the processes of waste elimination that lead to spiritual growth. Regardless of age, wealth, or wisdom, we are relatively powerless to alter the fact that we are at the mercy of a more powerful and transcendent power than the mere transitory power of men and institutions. History thoroughly and unequivocally bears this out.

Spiritual health keeps our entire being in balance. It provides healthy soil that can prevent us from being overweight and overbearing. Just as fruits and vegetables are the staples for supporting our physical health, unconditional love and forgiveness are the primary staples for supporting spiritual health. Peace, joy, humility and wisdom are the nuts, seeds, grains and legumes that round out a complete whole- food diet that supports our spiritual health.

As we develop a relationship with our Creator, we experience a new and improved body, mind, and spirit. As we selflessly share our newfound pearls of health and vitality with our neighbors, we improve our health, neighbors and planet. As expressed in the Holy Bible, the power of love, which is the life force of our spirit, can create a new heaven and a new earth, a place where the lion can coexist with the wolf and the lamb. The infant can play at the cobra's den and the child can place his hand in the viper's nest. Neither will be harmed nor destroyed because the world will be filled with the power of love.

Trusting in the supernatural power that created us enables the harmonious integration of body, mind, and spirit. The earthly goal of physical health, which is temporal, is transcended to spiritual health, which is eternal.

Important Health-promoting Items

The following are some of the health-promoting items that support an environment for optimum health at the spiritual level:

Acknowledgment of our Dependence on a Higher Power

Human beings are subject to the higher laws of nature, just like all phenomena in the universe. Recognition of our human boundaries opens our bodies and minds to superhuman healing forces. Acknowledgment of our dependence opens the pathways for us to achieve spiritual maturity. It is fascinating when we stop to think about the awesome complexity and balance of the universe. The more we explore and learn, the greater our appreciation for how much more there is to know. By following the laws of nature and trusting in the Creator that governs our universe, health is enabled beyond today's limited comprehension.

Love for our Fellow Man

Love is probably the most universal principle underlying most of our different belief systems. Love's mysterious healing energy uplifts us personally and improves our social relationships. It is powerful enough to "heal" our entire planet.

Daily Exercise of our Spirit

Practice makes perfect. It is important to regularly spend some quiet time for the awakening of our inner mind and spiritual self. Daily Bible study, prayer, and service to others are among the most powerful spiritual calisthenics known to man. With the daily distractions of today's frenetic pace, daily focus on our spiritual side will guard our immune system against the ever-increasing health challenges we face.

Learning from Nature

Nature teaches many lessons regarding nurturing and healthy living. By observing, studying and applying the powerful laws of nature to our lives, our spiritual enrichment will overcome the boundaries and mysteries of physical limitations.

An Active Prayer Life

Throughout history, civilizations have demonstrated their natural propensity to communicate with a higher power. Prayer is legendary for its powerful healing influences. Throughout our recorded history and still today, it heals many conditions with its powerfully effective life force. There are many things that may seem right in the light of human knowledge that in the end lead to disappointing results. An active prayer life opens our minds and hearts to the source of all knowledge, wisdom, and health.

Our spirit is what differentiates us from every other living thing on our planet. Many of us instinctively feed ourselves with the healing energy assimilated through the spirit. The spirit element is the most powerful element of our being which allows us to transcend the limitations of all known human knowledge to receive a mysteriously perfect and lasting gift of health.

I like to start all of my personalized health plans with the first and most important element, namely, "Spend special time in prayer daily. God can do everything and when we pray to Him, we can do everything He can do!"

Trust and reliance on a loving powerful God gives us the ability to enjoy a healthful lifestyle. Complete belief in God permits Him to fill our lives with *outrageous health.*

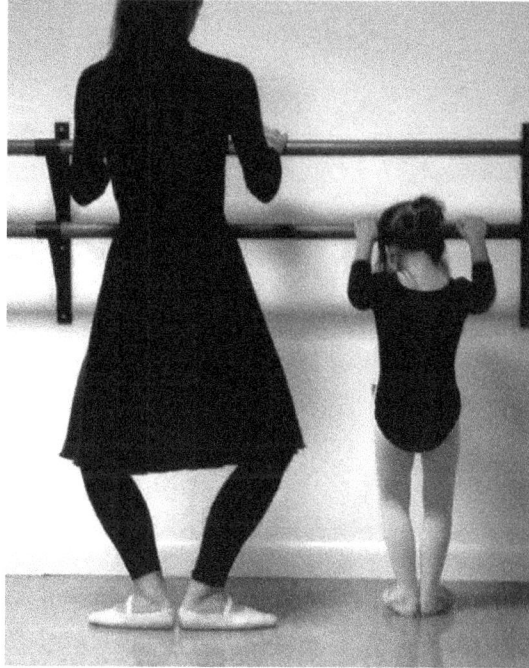

Moderation
and Balance

Moderation and balance are the underlying principles for all physical health factors. Although moderation is usually associated with avoiding harmful things like processed foods, caffeine, nicotine, alcohol, drugs and other waste elements. It also means moderation in things that are good. Overeating and poor combinations of good food, over-supplementation, indiscriminate use of eligible herbs and other specialized products, and improper amounts of exercise and rest can also compromise optimum physical health. Moderation means using good common sense. It provides the balance and self-control that permits the highest attainment of our physical, mental, and spiritual development.

With your Body, Mind, and Spirit harmoniously integrated, you will experience optimum and Total Health.

Moderation, balance, and self-control are necessary to avoid health-destroying behaviors. Alcohol, tobacco, and other drugs are enticing because they are promoted as fun, stimulating, and as a release from stress and pain. Even many innocent-appearing popular beverages contain drugs. Theophylline lurks in tea, and caffeine is hidden in most coffee and colas. Fruit-flavored wine coolers contain alcohol. Using alcohol, tobacco, and other drugs in any amount is hazardous because they may lead to addiction and harm. Some prescription drugs can be addictive, and they must be used with great caution and only when necessary. Drugs destroy purity of mind when they cause addiction; drugs destroy purity of soul when intoxication leads to abuse, inappropriate sex, or violent behavior. Drugs destroy purity of body when they cause disease and even death. Instead of artificial stimulants with a subsequent crash, get your highs from exercise. In place of chemical depressants and stimulants, get your relaxation from sunlight, water, and rest.

Moderation and balance are the underlying principles for all physical health factors. Although moderation is usually associated with avoiding harmful things like processed foods, caffeine, nicotine, alcohol, drugs, and other waste elements. It also means moderation in things that are good. Overeating and poor combinations of good food, over-supplementation, indiscriminate use of eligible herbs and other specialized products, and improper amounts of exercise and rest can also compromise optimum physical health. Moderation means using good common sense. It provides the balance and self-control that permits the highest attainment of our physical, mental, and spiritual development.

Temperance or moderation therefore means abstinence from things bad for us and moderation in things that are good. Is there any sense of moderation in the use of arsenic or strychnine? Definitely not! Some things are best totally avoided, things like tobacco, alcohol, and other dangerous addictive substances.

Problems with Alcohol Consumption

Alcohol is a legal yet addictive substance that we need to avoid totally. It is estimated that up to 15 percent of those who use alcohol will become either problem drinkers or actual alcoholics. Alcohol is a chemical compound known as ethyl alcohol, or ethanol that can be consumed in a beverage. There is a common belief that wine and beer are not nearly as damaging as hard liquor and mixed drinks. However, it is the amount of ethanol, regardless of where it came from that brings the adverse consequences. There is roughly half an ounce (15 grams) of pure ethanol in each of the following:

- 1 ounce of 80-proof liquor
- 5 ounces of wine
- 12 ounces of beer

The measurement of blood alcohol is expressed in milligrams (mg) per deciliter (dl) of blood.

80

Intoxication is correlated with the blood alcohol levels as follows:

Table 4. Intoxication Blood Alcohol Levels

<10 mg/dl (<0.01%)	no measurable intoxication
>10 mg/dl (>0.01%)	measurable intoxication
20 mg/dl (0.02%)	mellow feeling
50 mg /dl (0.05%)	social high
80 mg/dl (0.08 %)	reduced coordination (legal level of intoxication)
100 mg/dl (0.10%)	noticeably impaired coordination
200 mg/dl (0.20%)	confusion
300 mg/dl (0.30%)	loss of consciousness
>400 mg/dl (0.40%)	coma, death

Many people drink alcohol for its effects. These are a relaxation of the body, a loss of inhibitions, and an easing of aches and pains. These good feelings are a direct result of the blocking effect of alcohol on the frontal lobe of the brain, which is the seat of inhibition, reasoning, powers, memory, and judgment. As brain messages slow down, tensions seem to float away, and a person experiences a relaxed feeling. That is why alcohol is called the social lubricant.

In the stomach, the enzyme alcohol dehydrogenase, breaks down some 15 percent of ingested alcohol. The remaining 85 percent of the alcohol is converted in the liver. Females have less alcohol dehydrogenase than men; as a result, when a boy and a girl of the same weight are given equal amounts of alcohol, the girl will have a higher blood alcohol level than the boy. Females typically become more intoxicated on a given amount of alcohol than males. There are many side effects of alcohol consumption relating to the physical, emotional as well as social life:

- The immune system is damaged even by the social use of alcohol in the so- called "moderate drinker," increasing the risk of bacterial or viral infections. It takes only two drinks to reduce antibody production of B lymphocytes by 67 percent.

- Alcohol causes brain cells to die at an increased rate (alcoholic cerebellar degeneration and also cerebral dysfunction in the long term).

- Alcohol raises blood pressure (women seem to be more susceptible due to their relative lack of the enzyme alcohol dehydrogenase. As little as two or three drinks per day increase the risk of hypertension by 40 percent in women).

- Alcohol raises the risk of stroke (the famous Honolulu Heart Study found that even the so-called light drinkers of as little as 1–14 ounces per month have more than twice the risk of having one of these hemorrhagic strokes).

- Alcohol is clearly linked to several heart problems even though it is widely proclaimed that it is good for the heart (the high rate of sudden death among heavy alcohol users is likely due in part to dangerous heart rhythm disturbances; 20–30 percent of all cardiomyopathies in the U.S. is due to alcohol alone.)

- Alcohol is the leading cause of preventable mental retardation.

- Fetal Alcohol Syndrome, in which a woman consumes alcohol while pregnant, can negatively affect a fetus and/or infant in three major ways:

  1. A tendency to lag behind in physical growth both in the womb and after birth;

  2. Evidence of brain involvement with such problems as intellectual impairment, hyperactivity, distractibility, and impulsiveness;

  3. A characteristic set of facial abnormalities includes small eye openings, a small head circumference, a thin upper lip, skin folds at the corners of their eyes and a low nasal bridge.

There are many other problems related to alcohol. These help answer the question as to whether there is a need to drink or not. The answer is a resounding No! Government research reveals that alcohol causes more than 100,000 deaths per year in the U.S. Thus among drugs, alcohol is second only to tobacco as a cause of premature deaths in this nation, and is the third leading cause of death.

What about the evidence proclaimed by the media and medical journals that alcohol has positive cardiovascular health benefits for those who use it? It is generally accepted that alcohol is the mediator of some of these observed benefits. However, there are additional benefits from the flavonoids and other substances present in unfermented grape juice. Alcohol has been shown in observational studies to have some benefits. It is most important to note that the benefits were not observed in young people. The negative effects of alcohol are so significant, including the catastrophic risk of addiction, that experts do not recommend it. The editorials associated with the publication of such studies state that the risk-to-benefit ratio is not sufficient to warrant advising those who do not drink alcohol to start!

Problems with Tobacco Usage

Tobacco use is also a major and preventable cause of disease and premature death. It is responsible for nearly one in five deaths in the United States. It accounted for an estimated 430,700 premature deaths each year from 1990 to 1994 and more than $53 billion in direct medical costs in 1993. It now accounts for 5 million deaths per year worldwide!

Tobacco smoke has more than 4,800 chemicals; at least 69 are carcinogenic (cancer initiator). These include N-nitrosamine, polynuclear aromatic hydrocarbons, and other carcinogenic agents. There are at least 300 known poisons in tobacco smoke including nicotine, arsenic, radon, cyanide, phenol, DDT, asbestos, benzene, carbon monoxide, and formaldehyde. The three most harmful chemicals in cigarettes are nicotine, tar, and carbon monoxide.

There are more than 4,800 chemicals in tobacco smoke; at least 69 of them are carcinogenic (cancer initiator). These include N-nitrosamine, polynuclear aromatic hydrocarbons, and other carcinogenic agents. There are at least 300 known poisons in tobacco smoke including nicotine, arsenic, radon, cyanide, phenol, DDT, asbestos, benzene, carbon monoxide, and formaldehyde. The three most harmful chemicals in cigarettes are nicotine, tar, and carbon monoxide.

A number of chemicals in cigarette smoke have been linked to the formation of atherosclerosis (fatty deposits in the heart's blood vessel walls). The two most significant components are nicotine and carbon monoxide; nicotine damages the cells of the artery wall, allowing fatty substances from the blood to leak into the underlying tissues and start the process of atherosclerosis.

If blockage or narrowing of blood vessels takes place, a smoker may suffer from a variety of problems: hypertension, which is an elevation of blood pressure; aneurysm, or bulging of the aorta (the major blood vessel transporting blood from the heart to the rest of the body); and circulatory deficiencies. The individual will suffer from a shortage of oxygen to the heart; pain, called angina, may be experienced. Should the artery become totally blocked, a section of the heart is deprived of blood, a portion of heart muscle will die, and the individual will suffer a heart attack. This disease process is much more frequent in smokers.

If obstruction takes place in the blood vessels of the brain, then the patient may suffer a stroke. It can be either ischemic (blood supply to the brain is cut off) or hemorrhagic (blood vessel bursts, preventing a normal flow and allowing blood to leak into an area of the brain and destroy it). Because nerves in the brain cross over to the opposite side of the body, symptoms appear on the side of the body opposite the damaged side of the brain.

Carbon monoxide (CO) accelerates the development of atherosclerosis; and, it has other widespread damaging effects. Once the hemoglobin in the red blood cells binds with carbon monoxide, the capacity to carry oxygen is diminished. All the cells in the body, including those of a fetus (when present), are relatively deprived of oxygen. The immune defenses of smokers are lowered, and they may suffer from a variety of problems ranging from influenza to cancers in sites other than the respiratory tract in which disease would normally be eliminated by an adequately functioning immune system.

Cigarette smoking is a contributing factor for several other cancers. There are many other problems caused by smoking, such as:

- Headaches, which may be the result of carbon monoxide as well as decreased cerebral blood flow to the brain

- Influenza, at a rate of 3 times more than non-smokers because of lowered immunity and inactivation of local protective mechanisms

- A degree of infertility in both females and males.

- Bronchitis and emphysema

- Premature aging

- Halitosis (foul breath), which is unresponsive to mouthwash and toothpaste

- Gingivitis, an inflammation of the gums resulting in a three-fold greater loss of teeth than that of non-smokers

- Dental cavities, which are three times more common in smokers because of increased plaque, bacterial growth, and decay.

True temperance is not only avoiding the use of these drugs because they destroy our health but also to use in moderation the healthful things, such as:

- Sleep. Too much sleep is detrimental to your health. E.C. Hammond discovered the lowest death rate was in those men averaging around 7–8 hours of sleep per night, whereas those who either skimped on their sleep or spent too much time sleeping in bed, died at a younger age than those who enjoyed the proper amount of sleep regularly.

- Sunshine. Though a source of vitamin D, excess sunlight can become a cancer-promoting agent.

- Moderate exercise. This is vital for optimum health; however, excessive exercise to the point of exhaustion, which is seen typically in some athletes, can have a negative effect.

- Sexual activity. Though a God-given gift, is often abused.

- Food. Though essential, it may be taken in excess, resulting in obesity. When restricted abnormally, it can result in deficiencies.

Therefore, practice moderation and balance in all things, avoiding all things that are harmful – legal drugs like alcohol and tobacco, all illicit drugs, unnecessary prescription drug and; harmful food choices. Instead, practice God-given self-control, in all healthful practices.

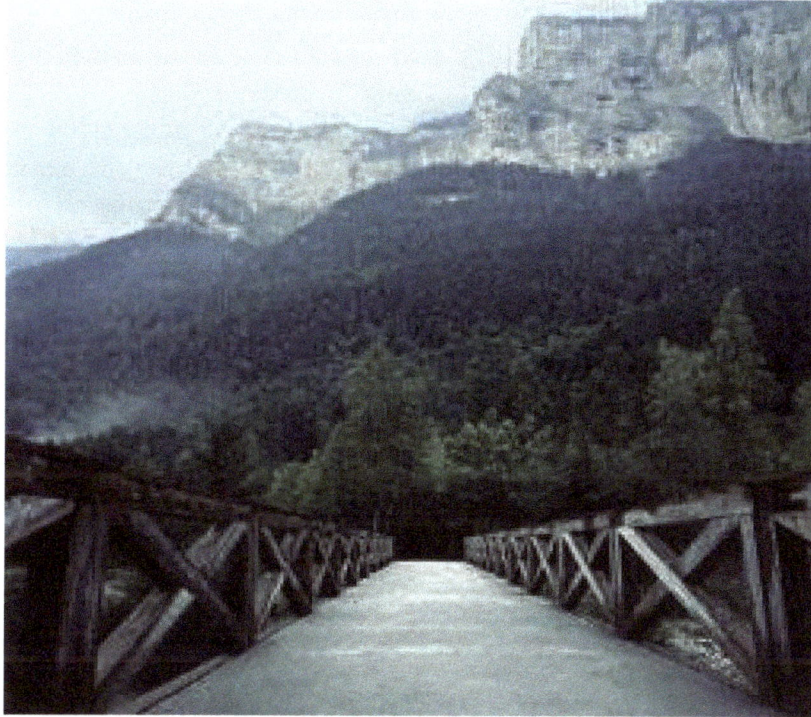

Making the Transition to a Healthier Lifestyle

Individual Responsibility

Total health requires personal responsibility. We are all individuals with unique capacities and requirements. These guidelines are offered as a blueprint, not a standard solution. They can be applied as they fit individual needs and capacities. It is important to have a basic understanding of how your body works and what is best for you based on your lifestyle, activity level, genetic predisposition, and desired health goals. Many of the stressful effects on your body should be understood and avoided as much as possible. It is important to learn, develop a well-thought-out health plan, and then put it into practice. The guidelines provided are not a prescription. They should be used as a guide to develop your own personalized health strategy.

You own your health, so, you have enormous latitude in choosing the strategy for optimizing your personalized, dietary regimen. Certainly, this does not mean that everyone has to become a nutritionist or health professional. It is important, however, to develop a basic understanding of body functions and nutritional requirements. Once armed with this understanding, you may even opt to work with a qualified health practitioner or practitioners who are sympathetic to meeting your requirements.

The more skills and strategies you have available, the greater your opportunity for reaching your desired health goals through proper nutrition. If you hire a carpenter to build a house, you are much more likely to have your expectations and requirements met if the carpenter has a full complement of tools as opposed to just a hammer and a pair of pliers. The Hierarchy of Nutrients clearly demonstrates that our bodies perform best with fruits, vegetables, nuts, seeds, etc. All other foods are tolerated based on our individual requirements and capacities. Common sense tells us that we should honor these principles in accordance with our desired physical, mental, emotional, and spiritual goals.

Making the Transition

Care must be taken when making a transition from a compromised lifestyle to a more holistic and integrated health program. When your body undergoes major changes in a short period of time, it can often experience discomfort. We often crave the things to which we have become addicted. Your body, however, becomes addicted to good habits just as it does to poor health practices. It will take time to reprogram your habits and lifestyle.

The discomfort a person generally feels during a lifestyle transition is sometimes referred to as a "healing crisis." Your body always strives to improve, repair, and continually cleanse itself. Given a new healthful environment, your body tends to release stored waste and repair metabolic systems at a faster rate than the elimination organs can handle. Feelings of nausea, headaches, light-headedness, and flu-like aches and pains are not uncommon. It is important to understand this phenomenon and work through it to a healthful conclusion. Working with these discomforts while you employ the appropriate nutritional and support strategies will yield significant benefits. These symptoms are part of the balancing process necessary for optimum health.

For major changes in diet, strong motivation and willpower may be required. In many instances a more gradual change may be pursued to avoid or minimize the healing crisis. You may incorporate changes in "bite-sized" pieces. Even by doing this, you will make significant progress in a reasonable period of time. It is important to remember that a changed diet and lifestyle does not occur overnight. It will take some time to reclaim your optimum health. It could take from a few months to several years for major improvements to occur. Your body improves in cycles with plateaus of health followed by short periods of waste-elimination symptoms and conditions. Each plateau gets progressively longer and the elimination conditions become shorter and milder.

There are several aids, like drinking distilled water, fasting, colon hydrotherapy, juicing, short-term cleansing diets, and related strategies that can assist in making the transition to healthy lifestyle practices. Health practitioners and educators with an understanding of natural healing principles can provide valuable support during lifestyle transitions. A couple of books referenced at the end of this book offer some practical approaches to making dietary transitions. These include McDougal's, The McDougal Program and Boutenko's, 12 Steps to Raw Foods. Investing in your personal health development and maintenance will repay you attractive dividends. Prayer is a very powerful enabler in any dietary or lifestyle program. God can do everything, and when we pray to Him, He will assist us in our efforts because He desires for us to be in good health, which is one of His greatest blessings.

How to Eat Right

One of the most important factors in maximizing the nourishment we receive is how we eat. The physiology of digestion is not well understood by many health professionals. Yet, it plays a very important role in promoting health and minimizing degenerative disease processes. The following list of dietary guidelines will help you get the most out of the foods you eat.

Chew Foods Slowly and Thoroughly

Chewing food slowly and thoroughly prepares the entire digestive system for its job of breaking down food into basic nutrients. Carbohydrate food digestion begins with enzymes in the mouth. Protein chewed in the mouth is broken down into more manageable pieces for the stomach, and fats chewed in the mouth trigger both pancreatic and liver enzyme processes. Chewing starts the initial breakdown of food, while activating the muscle, nerve, and enzymatic processes required for digestion. Food should always be eaten in manageable bites and chewed slowly. Even liquids (which should not be taken with meals) should be thoroughly mixed with the saliva in the mouth. A good practice to ensure adequate salivation of both foods and liquids is to "drink your foods and chew your liquids."

Take No Liquids with Meals

Liquids, preferably water, should be taken between meals (at least 1/2 hour after fruit meals, 2 to 4 hours after more complex meals). Taking liquids with meals tends to dilute the digestive juices. The liquid must be absorbed before solid food digestion can take place. This delay in digestion can lead to food fermentation and putrefaction. In most instances, very cold and very hot liquids should be avoided. Cold liquids retard digestion until the stomach can warm them sufficiently. They also can shock and bring about spasms in the internal organs. Chronic use of hot liquids can weaken the nerves and digestion system.

Allow 4 to 6 Hours Between Meals

The stomach needs 3 to 4 hours to finish its work and should rest for an hour or two in order to be recharged for the next meal. This will help avoid both stomach and intestinal ailments. It is best to have nothing between meals. Having allergies and being underweight or overweight are among the many problems that are common among snackers. By allowing a minimum of 4 to 6 hours between meals you should be able to completely digest your food and rest the digestive system before the next meal. Dinner should be light and eaten early.

Incomplete breakdown of foods occurs because of the slower digestion of foods eaten in the evening, especially right before sleep. The fermentation resulting from this practice increases the buildup of waste in the blood, causes several ailments, and interrupts restful sleep. Fruits, vegetables, and moderate amounts of complex carbohydrates empty from the stomach faster than heavier foods like fat, protein and complex cooked foods; therefore, they are ideal dinner foods.

Eat in a Relaxed Environment

To ensure proper digestion, take the time to relax and make your stomach comfortable prior to eating your meal. Eating should take place when you are not emotionally or physically stressed. Eating to soothe abdominal discomfort only perpetuates and worsens gastrointestinal problems.

Be Temperate and Balanced

Temperance and balance are the underlying principles for all physical health factors. Temperance is usually associated with avoiding harmful things like processed foods, caffeine, nicotine, alcohol, drugs, and waste elements. Temperance also means moderation in things that are good. Overeating and poor combinations of good food, over-supplementation, and indiscriminate use of edible herbs and other specialized products can also compromise optimum physical health. We will discuss principles and guidelines for this important topic in the next section on the ideal diet. Temperance means using good common sense. It provides the balance and self- control that permits the highest attainment of our physical, mental, and spiritual development.

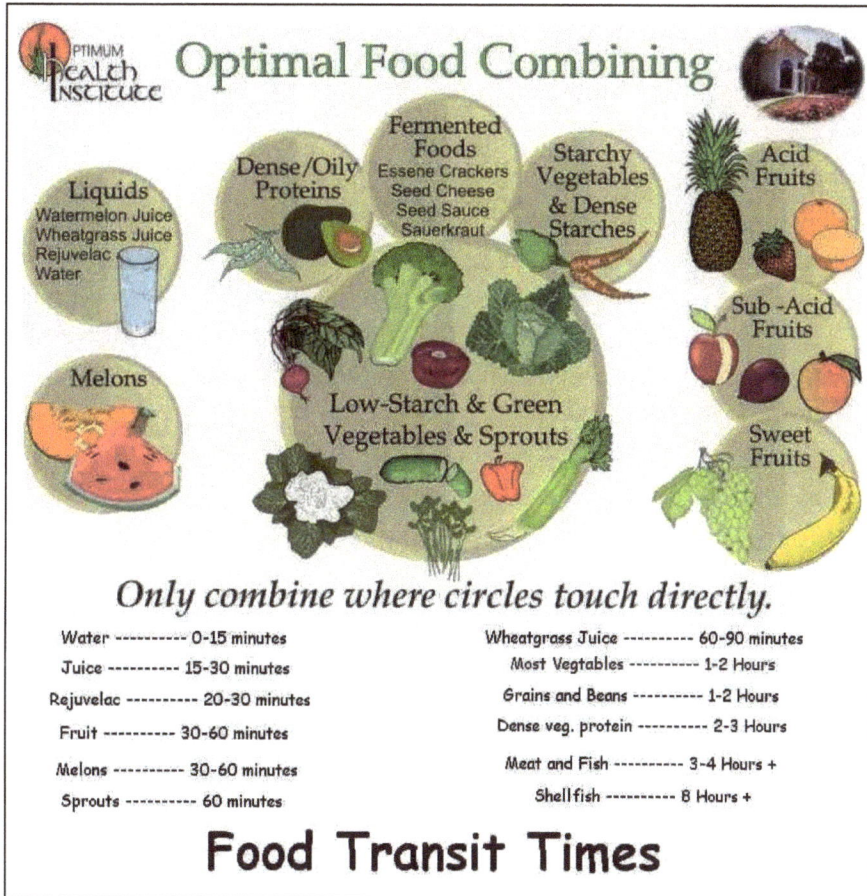

Optimal Food Combining

Liquids
Watermelon Juice
Wheatgrass Juice
Rejuvelac
Water

Melons

Dense/Oily Proteins

Fermented Foods
Essene Crackers
Seed Cheese
Seed Sauce
Sauerkraut

Starchy Vegetables & Dense Starches

Low-Starch & Green Vegetables & Sprouts

Acid Fruits

Sub-Acid Fruits

Sweet Fruits

Only combine where circles touch directly.

Water ---------- 0-15 minutes	Wheatgrass Juice ---------- 60-90 minutes
Juice ---------- 15-30 minutes	Most Vegtables ---------- 1-2 Hours
Rejuvelac ---------- 20-30 minutes	Grains and Beans ---------- 1-2 Hours
Fruit ---------- 30-60 minutes	Dense veg. protein ---------- 2-3 Hours
Melons ---------- 30-60 minutes	Meat and Fish ---------- 3-4 Hours +
Sprouts ---------- 60 minutes	Shellfish ---------- 8 Hours +

Food Transit Times

Proper Food Combining

It is not necessary to get every type of food (fruit, vegetable, nuts, seeds, proteins, carbohydrates, etc.) at every meal. Your body needs these nutrients over a reasonable period of time during the day for complete and balanced nourishment and function.

All the animals on our planet eat one food at a time. And, our digestive system works best when it works on one type of food at a time. However, there are compatible combinations of foods that optimize digestion. Proper food combining maintains this delicate balance while meeting the need for both variety and simplicity in our diets. Proper food combining provides for optimum nutrient availability and ease of digestion.

For those on a very good natural food diet with well-balanced metabolic function, food combining may be unnecessary. On the other hand, for those with weaker digestive systems or as an aid to minimize overeating a complex diet of rich foods, food combining can offer significant digestive support.

The earliest commentary on this important topic that I am aware of dates back to the mid-1800s and appears in Ellen G. White's landmark book, Counsels on Diets and Foods. The principles of food combining were first explained in the early 1900s by John Tilden, M.D., and William Hay, M.D. In the middle 1900s, Herbert Shelton, N.D., devoted 50 years to the study of food combining and wrote Food Combining Made Easy.

Food combining concerns the physiology of digestion. The digestive system has a large number of secreting glands that are responsible for breaking down the foods we eat. The content and timing of digestive secretions determine the thoroughness and efficiency within which ingested foods are broken down for cellular metabolism. The purpose of breaking down foods is to provide the basic elements that feed the cells of our body; namely, simple sugars, amino acids, fatty acids, vitamins, and minerals. Complex and incompatible food combinations of even the most nutritious foods may significantly impact the thoroughness and effectiveness of their breakdown for cellular nourishment. This is a problem particularly for persons who chronically overeat and/or have weak digestive systems.

The digestive system is marvelously engineered to handle any single, whole, and natural food. Even though whole foods in their natural state contain a combination of proteins, fats, and carbohydrates, the digestive system is designed to handle both the timing and content of digestive juices to break down whole foods into simpler nutrients. When several different types of food are taken together, however, efficient digestion may be challenged to the point of causing "indigestion" and thereby compromising the attainment of optimum nutritional value from our foods. This problem is made worse by overly manipulated, richly combined, overcooked, processed, and unnatural foods. The results of poor food combining can be the expenditure of large amounts of digestive energy, fermentation, putrefaction, and lowered nutrient availability. Chronic, poor food combinations can lead to several degenerative disease processes as a consequence of diminished nutrient support and accumulated waste.

On the other hand, the benefits of proper food combining are more thorough and complete digestion, better energy conservation for the digestive system, and higher nutrient availability to our cells and tissues.

For practical purposes, most people do not eat single foods. This is where a basic understanding of proper food combining can help in making the most prudent food choices.

General Food Combining Tips

The Food Combining Chart, food combination examples later in this section, and the practical meal examples in the Appendix should be consulted to better understand the application of the following food combination guidelines:

Meals Should Contain No More than 3 or 4 Compatible Foods

Limiting the number of foods eaten at each meal will lessen the burden on the digestive system and improve the digestibility of your meals. The more complex the food combinations are, the more energy and time required for complete breakdown. The Food Combining Chart at the end of this section demonstrates compatible food combinations.

Fruits Should Generally Be Eaten Alone

Fruits are extremely efficient and provide very high nutrient value. They are rich in enzymes that render them predigested and therefore require little to no digestion in the stomach. Their digestion is completed in the small intestine, and the nutrients are immediately available to nourish your body. Since fruits require a short amount of time in the stomach, they combine poorly with most starchy, protein, and vegetable foods (that require extended digestive times) and tend to ferment when eaten with or after these foods.

Some fruits combine poorly even with each other. Fruits fall into three main categories: acid, sub-acid and sweet. The Food Combining Chart shows the most compatible combinations.

Note: Melons are a special case, and should be eaten alone for best results.

Eat No More than One Concentrated Food per Meal

For best results, meals should be planned around one concentrated food type. Select your main course from the grain, starch, or protein family of foods. You can include one or two vegetables and a raw vegetable salad as a practical application of this guideline.

Carbohydrate-rich Foods Combine Poorly with Protein-rich Foods

All carbohydrate digestion begins in the mouth with the enzyme amylase (ptyalin). Thorough chewing mixes this enzyme with food and begins the breakdown of carbohydrates in the mouth, a process that continues in the stomach and small intestine. Stomach secretions optimized for breaking down carbohydrates are more alkaline, while stomach secretions optimized for breaking down concentrated protein foods are more acidic.

When both concentrated carbohydrates and proteins are included in the same meal, the resulting secretions may be unable to break down either food thoroughly. This compromised situation results in an incomplete breakdown of both types of food and can lead to the fermentation of carbohydrates and putrefaction of the protein foods, which leads to poor nutrient absorption and waste accumulation.

Most Vegetables Combine Well with Either Carbohydrates or Proteins

Vegetables are rich in enzymes and nutrients that complement complex carbohydrate and protein foods. The rich variety of vegetables greatly improves the practical application of proper food combining for nutrient-rich meals.

Fats Combine Poorly with Proteins

Fats inhibit the production of stomach secretions required for thorough protein breakdown. Fats tend to combine well with both vegetables and starches but should be eaten in moderation.

Acid Foods Combine Poorly with Carbohydrate and Protein Foods

Acid foods, like vinegar and various pickled foods, tend to inhibit the production of both amylase (ptyalin) and pepsin, two important enzymes for carbohydrate and protein breakdown, respectively. These types of foods also provide little to no nutritional value to your body.

Refined Sugar Combines Poorly with Both Carbohydrates and Proteins

Refined sugar retards amylase (ptyalin) and the production of secretions in the stomach. Its digestion takes place in the small intestines and tends to ferment when kept in the stomach for even short periods of time, causing indigestion and other harmful gastrointestinal problems. On the other hand, sugar in its natural state, as in fruits or sugar cane, digests extremely well.

Milk Combines Poorly with Most Foods

If used at all, milk should be eaten alone and should be raw certified milk (which is difficult to find). Milk is a very concentrated food that is high in fat and protein. It starts as a liquid, but curdles and turns into a solid once it enters your stomach. This interferes with both protein and carbohydrate digestion. The worst combinations with milk are fish, meat and eggs.

Pasteurization further compromises the digestibility of milk. This process destroys important enzymes required for the breakdown of the protein and lactose sugar for effective utilization by your body. Milk is highly acidic and mucous-forming. There are several popular milk substitute products currently on the market, which also require careful evaluation for their overall nutritional value. Many are processed and 'fortified' to the point of marginal nutritional value. Homemade nut, soy, and whole grain milks are safer and more nutritious alternatives.

Processed and Meat-substitute "Vegetarian" Foods Combine Poorly

Modern food technology has produced many combinations that are foreign to the gastrointestinal system. They confuse your body since they are generally non-foods that are deficient in balanced nutrients, lack important enzymes, and contain harmful preservatives and additives. Your body can easily handle small amounts of these non-foods. However, the cumulative effect of combinations of these foods can be stressful. Compromise of the immune system in fighting off the effects of these non-foods and several degenerative disease processes are often the result of continued reliance on these food sources.

Exceptions

The above principles are general guidelines and are not meant to be hard and fast rules. One's individual capacity is the best judge of the appropriateness of food combining. As with most things, there are exceptions to these guidelines. For example:

- Cellulose and fruits with fatty oils (such as apples and avocados) and sun- dried fruit (such as figs, dates, and raisins) tend to combine favorably with fresh raw vegetables in salads.
- Celery, cucumber, and lettuce combine well with most fruits.
- Fruit vegetables, like avocados and tomatoes, tend to function as vegetables.
- Nuts and seeds tend to combine well with most fruits.

The following basic principles help simplify putting together meals using the above food-combining principles:

1. Decide what concentrated food you would like to eat (protein or carbohydrate-based food) and include compatible combinations of vegetables
2. Fruit should generally be eaten alone. Even when combining fruits, it is generally best to avoid combining the more acidic fruits, like pineapples and oranges, with the sweet fruits, like bananas, figs and dates.
3. Nuts and seeds tend to combine well with most fruits and salad greens.

The examples and charts on the following pages provide additional help in putting together nutritious and well-combined meals.

While little is taught in traditional health institutions and insufficient studies are available to date, those wishing to maximize nutrient bioavailability and minimize waste accumulations are encouraged to investigate and evaluate the role of proper food combining in their personalized health program. Most will realize surprisingly positive digestive and overall health-enhancing results.

Eat proteins and carbohydrates at separate meals
Eat only one concentrated protein at each meal
Treat juices, fruit or vegetable, as a whole food

Take milk alone or not at all
Desert Desserts
Cold food, including liquids, inhibit digestion

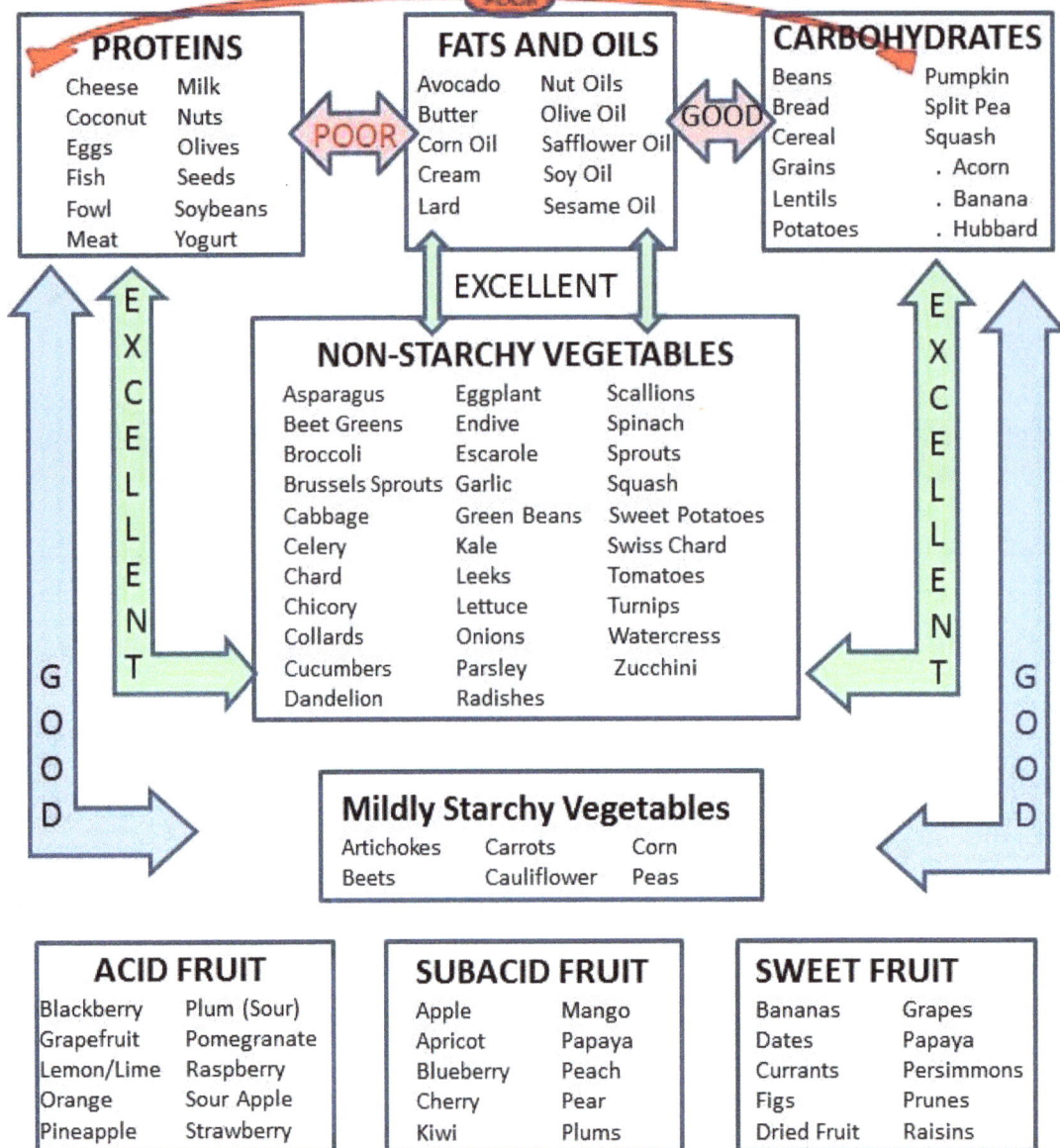

POOR

PROTEINS

Cheese	Milk
Coconut	Nuts
Eggs	Olives
Fish	Seeds
Fowl	Soybeans
Meat	Yogurt

POOR

FATS AND OILS

Avocado	Nut Oils
Butter	Olive Oil
Corn Oil	Safflower Oil
Cream	Soy Oil
Lard	Sesame Oil

GOOD

CARBOHYDRATES

Beans	Pumpkin
Bread	Split Pea
Cereal	Squash
Grains	. Acorn
Lentils	. Banana
Potatoes	. Hubbard

EXCELLENT

E X C E L L E N T

E X C E L L E N T

NON-STARCHY VEGETABLES

Asparagus	Eggplant	Scallions
Beet Greens	Endive	Spinach
Broccoli	Escarole	Sprouts
Brussels Sprouts	Garlic	Squash
Cabbage	Green Beans	Sweet Potatoes
Celery	Kale	Swiss Chard
Chard	Leeks	Tomatoes
Chicory	Lettuce	Turnips
Collards	Onions	Watercress
Cucumbers	Parsley	Zucchini
Dandelion	Radishes	

GOOD

GOOD

Mildly Starchy Vegetables

Artichokes	Carrots	Corn
Beets	Cauliflower	Peas

ACID FRUIT

Blackberry	Plum (Sour)
Grapefruit	Pomegranate
Lemon/Lime	Raspberry
Orange	Sour Apple
Pineapple	Strawberry

SUBACID FRUIT

Apple	Mango
Apricot	Papaya
Blueberry	Peach
Cherry	Pear
Kiwi	Plums

SWEET FRUIT

Bananas	Grapes
Dates	Papaya
Currants	Persimmons
Figs	Prunes
Dried Fruit	Raisins

Eat fruit alone as a meal
Fruits should not be eaten between meals
while other food is digesting

Do not eat sweet fruits with acid fruits
It is best to eat melons alone not even with other
fruits

Figure 3. Food Combining Chart

Using The Food Combining Chart

Food Type	Combines Well with	Combines Poorly with
Acid Fruits	Other Acid Fruits, Sub-acid Fruits	Sweet Fruits, Proteins, Vegetables, Carbohydrates
Sub-acid Fruits	All Fruits	Proteins, Vegetables, Carbohydrates
Sweet Fruits	Other Sweet Fruits, Sub-acid Fruits	Acid Fruits, Proteins, Vegetables, Carbohydrates
All Fruits	Lettuce, Celery, Cucumbers, Nuts, Seeds	Most Other Foods
Melons	Other Melons	Proteins, Vegetables, Carbohydrates
Proteins	Non-Starchy Vegetables	All Fruits, Starchy Vegetables, Carbohydrates
Vegetables	Proteins, Carbohydrates	All Fruits
Carbohydrates	All Vegetables	Proteins, All Fruits
Nuts/Seeds	Acid fruits, Non-starchy Vegetables	Most Other Foods
Milk	Itself	Most Other Foods

Food Combining Examples

Good Combination Examples	Poor Combination Examples
Oranges, pineapple, strawberry, grapes	Oranges, bananas, figs
Cereal w/ rice milk, whole wheat toast	Cereal with any fruit or milk
Fruit 1/2 hr. before cereal	Fruit after cereal
Fruit salad with nuts or seeds	Fruit salad with any meal
Rice, corn, vegetables, salad	Rice and beans and chicken
Beans, green vegetables, salad	Beans, rice, salad, fruit
Potatoes, any vegetables, salad	Potatoes, vinegar w/salad, fruit
Whole grains, vegetables, salad	Veggie burger, salad, fruit
Vegetable soup, salad	Soup, white bread, fruit
Salad with olive oil, lemon, garlic/onions	Salad with oil and vinegar
Salad with nut or vegetable dressing	Salad with commercial dressings
Fig, date, banana juice	Orange, banana, carrot juice

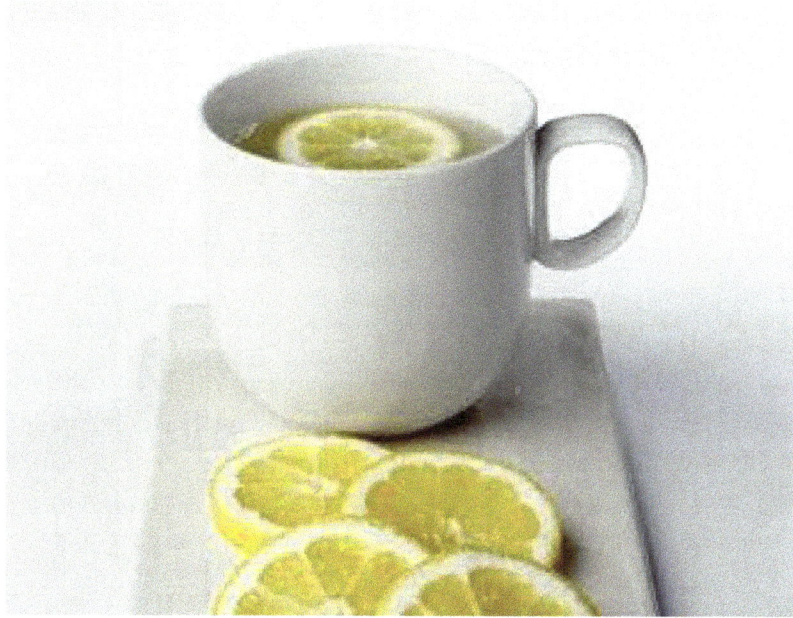

Eliminating Waste from the Body

In the beginning of this book we referred to a formula for physical health that promoted a balance between maximizing nourishment and minimizing waste retention. The previous sections provided guidelines for maximizing nourishment. Here we will review some guidelines for minimizing waste retention.

To the extent that you practice good dietary and lifestyle habits, you support the processes for waste elimination from your body. There are seven elimination systems or organs in your body: the lungs, skin, kidneys, colon, liver, bladder, and lymphatic system. Any blockage or compromised function in any of these systems will compromise the attainment of optimum health. A diet rich in foods with a high water content (fruits and vegetables), sufficient pure water, and simple, properly combined foods significantly enhance the elimination of waste from your body.

Recommended regimens for various ways to eliminate body waste are provided below. They are general recommendations only. It is suggested that you seek the advice of a naturopath or other qualified health professional to execute the fast that is best for your body. For instance, with the gall bladder/liver flush, a diabetic or pre-diabetic would be concerned with sugar/insulin levels. In this flush, it may be appropriate to reduce the daily amount of apple juice normally recommended and juice celery, cucumber, and lettuce along with the apples, and to add light, vegetable rice soups and salads.

Elimination Aids

There are several aids like drinking distilled water, fasting, colon hydrotherapy, juicing, short-term cleansing diets and related strategies that can assist in making the transition to healthy lifestyle practices. Health practitioners and educators with an understanding of natural healing principles can provide valuable support for lifestyle transitions. The investment in your personal health development and maintenance will repay you attractive dividends. The following are some important aids to eliminating accumulated waste from your body.

Distilled Water

Distilled water is the purest form of water for your body. Distilled water is free of inorganic minerals and metals and is excellent for the removal of harmful substances from your body. Fruit contains the highest amount and highest quality of distilled water. Other options available as purified water sources include water treated with reverse osmosis, deionization, charcoal filtration, and ozonization. However, steam distillation tends to be the best for eliminating 100 percent of all bacterial and viral organisms and other non-gaseous metal and mineral impurities.

Exercise

Exercise engages the lymphatic system, increases circulation, and mobilizes several metabolic functions. When perspiration is induced, elimination is encouraged through the largest eliminatory organ, the skin. When used in moderation, based on individual needs and capacities, exercise provides dynamic and powerful waste elimination for your body and mind.

Massage

Most massage techniques engage muscular and other movements throughout your body, which encourages the elimination of waste from your tissues and muscles. Several massage techniques have good results in cleansing the lymphatic system. Deep tissue, Rolfing, neuromuscular massage and related techniques help to restore structural and functional integrity, while performing beneficial waste mobilization and elimination. Reflexology, in the form of hand and foot massages, is an example of a technique that can be self-administered.

Liver/Gallbladder and Kidney Flushes

There are several dietary, juicing, and herbal strategies that help flush the kidneys and liver of waste overloads. Watermelon, whole or in juice form, is one of many kidney flushes that can be used. Herbs such as juniper berries, uva ursi, and buchu root also promote the flushing of your kidneys. The liver/gallbladder flush is a very powerful and effective strategy for support of your body's ability to flush out your liver. A liver/gallbladder flush consists of:

- 3 to 5 days of organic, unrefined apple juice
- Cleansing herbs (e.g., cascara sagrada, turkey rhubarb, etc.)
- Ending on the last day with 2 to 4 ounces of cold pressed virgin olive oil blended with the juice of 1 lemon.
- Lie down on your right side for at least 1/2 hour after drinking the olive oil and lemon juice blend.

Variations of the liver/gallbladder flush use combinations of grapefruit, orange, and lemon juice blended with varying levels of olive oil, based on tolerance and level of flushing desired.

Colon Hydrotherapy

Colon hydrotherapy is the gentle filling of the large intestines with warm, purified or filtered water for the elimination of accumulated waste, and for stimulation and tonification (encourages gentle peristalsis) of the colon. Cleansing of the colon relieves the burden of elimination from the other eliminatory systems and provides therapeutic support in the protection against a variety of degenerative conditions and diseases. It allows more waste to be eliminated from your entire body.

Fasting, Juicing, and Cleansing Herbs

There are several techniques and programs incorporating fasting, juicing, and cleansing herbs that support waste elimination and contribute to a wide range of therapeutic results. Care should be taken to ensure proper use of these techniques. Indiscriminate and improper use of these approaches, especially with some popular cleansing herbs, can have undesirable results. Proper use of these cleansing approaches has a very powerful therapeutic effect on a wide range of conditions, ailments, and diseases.

Fasting is the most powerful and dynamic cleansing and healing technique. True fasting consists of drinking only water in an environment of complete physiological and mental rest. When fasting is not practical, several intermediary approaches, e.g., fruit and/or vegetable juicing programs and the Master Cleanse program, can be pursued. The Master Cleanse program consists of pure distilled water plus the following:

- 2 tablespoons of fresh lemon juice per 8 ounces of water
- 1–2 tablespoons of organic, grade B maple syrup per 8 ounces of water
- A pinch of cayenne pepper per 8 ounces of water.

Various parasite, worm, and related elimination herbal protocols can also be effective, when appropriately used. The purpose of these treatments is to rid the body of harmful organisms that can compromise the body's ability to effectively eliminate waste and restore itself to optimum health. It is advisable to work with a qualified health professional or person knowledgeable in the physiological aspects of fasting and cleansing programs for optimum results.

Deep Breathing

There are several deep breathing techniques that have a powerful cleansing effect on the blood, cells, and lungs. Note that exhaling is the part of deep breathing that provides waste elimination. Most asthmatics have problems breathing out, which is the major cause of the wheezing and asthma attack process. In your deep breathing exercises, start slowly at a count of four for the inhalation and try to exhale at a count of one and one half to two times the inhale, six or eight. This should be done without straining. Increase the count to your capacity and comfort level. Deep breathing techniques can also be very relaxing and cleansing to the mind and spirit.

Skin and Tongue Brushing

Skin brushing with a long-handled vegetable-bristled brush removes loose dead skin from your body; it also stimulates the skin and other underlying processes, and aids lymphatic elimination. Skin brushing should be done top to bottom for the upper body and bottom to top for the lower extremities. The strokes should be circular and toward the intestinal area for both the upper and lower parts of your body.

Tongue brushing removes waste eliminated through the tongue, cleans the breath, and may stimulate important reflex points that affect the entire body.

Avoiding Environmental Toxins

In addition to avoiding harmful preservatives and additives in foods, food processing, and food preparation, there are many household, neighborhood, and workplace toxins that should be avoided and eliminated to relieve the eliminatory burdens of your body. These include certain personal hygiene and grooming products, cleaning products, and chemicals, lawn and garden products, poor ventilation and fumes, metal fillings in the teeth, excessive exposure to radiation, chlorinated and fluoridated water, and over-the-counter pharmaceuticals. This is a very important area, which is covered in more detail in several reference books listed at the end of this book. Taking proper care can offer substantial benefits in minimizing the waste accumulated from a variety of sources including polluted air, tap water, the foods we eat, and other controllable and uncontrollable environmental factors.

Summary

Health, wellness, nutrition, and proper diet are broad and comprehensive topics. The more you learn, the more you appreciate and are humbled by the complexities and the simplicity of realizing total health. Achieving and maintaining good dietary practices involves other topics not covered here, which will require further study. However, you will find these guidelines useful in understanding many of the basics of optimum health. The selected bibliography and appendices provide additional information on related topics, which will assist the serious student in developing a personalized dietary philosophy and strategy.

The preceding practical and basic guidelines are offered, not as a prescription, but as a guide or framework for basic dietary considerations. Health and overall systemic wellness are achieved through the right balance of dietary factors to meet individual needs and capacities. Food and diet clearly play a pivotal role but must be accompanied by other lifestyle factors to achieve optimum health and vitality.

Nature is the best guide for optimal food consumption to support dietary requirements. From nature we receive the most important foods in the most abundant supply and the most available form for our consumption. In order of importance, the priorities for human consumption are air, water, sunlight, fruits, vegetables, nuts, seeds, grains, legumes, and then flesh and dairy foods. All processed, manufactured, canned and packaged foods are junk foods. The greater the consumption of pure, clean foods based on nature's formula (raw, whole foods, as close to the way nature provides them, as practical), the better the odds of attaining naturally superior health.

Health at the mind and spiritual levels also requires nourishment. An open mind supplemented with a loving heart sets the foundation for health at these levels.

Accumulated waste must also be eliminated for optimum health. Nourishment and waste elimination provide a balanced environment for harmoniously integrating the body, mind, and spirit for the attainment of total health.

Total health through diet cannot be forced on us. It is up to each of us to freely pursue the best choices from the options available. Proper diet plays a pivotal role in helping us achieve the harmonious integration of our body, mind, and spirit. It is an important enabler for experiencing **Total Health!**

**May you continue to receive God's richest blessings as
you pursue your endeavors for achieving Total Health!**

Apendix A:
Health Quotient (HQ),
a simple health evaluation tool

Instructions for using the Health Quotient (HQ)

For each item indicate how often you do each item. If never or rarely (1–3 times a month), enter a zero; if sometimes (1–2 days a week), enter a 3; if most of the time (4 or more times a week), enter a 6; if daily (6 or 7 days a week), then enter a 10. Total both scores and subtract the Factors Minimizing Health from the Factors Maximizing Health. The result is your HQ.

It is possible to get a negative score (factors minimizing health outweigh the factors maximizing health). A maximum HQ of 150 would indicate superior health. A score of 100–125 should be a good intermediary goal for most of us. A score of 60–100 represents sub-optimum health even though there may be no current symptoms. A score of less than 60 will be problematic for most people and requires improvement. By looking at both the positive and negative elements relating to health, you can make some practical adjustments to meet your personal health objectives.

SCORING	POINTS
Never/Rarely	0
Sometimes	3
Most of the time	6
Daily	10

This is just a simple HQ applying the simple formula to basic health and wellness principles.

Try it, apply it, have fun with it and enjoy

Good Health!

FACTORS MAXIMIZING HEALTH	SCORE	FACTORS MINIMIZING HEALTH	SCORE
1. Plant Foods (Fruits, Veggies, Nuts, Seeds)	____	Flesh Foods	____
2. Chew Food Slowly and Thoroughly	____	Meat Substitutes	____
3. Avoid Liquids with Meals	____	Fried Foods	____
4. 4 To 6 Hours between Meals	____	Recreational Drugs	____
5. Small Supper at Least 3 Hrs. before Bed	____	Prescription Drugs	____
6. Sufficient Water	____	Dairy Products	____
7. Deep Breathing	____	Alcoholic Beverages	____
8. Exercise	____	Tobacco	____
9. Sufficient Sunlight When Available	____	Caffeine or Chocolate	____
10. Sufficient Rest (6 – 9 hours)	____	Excessive Work or Exercise	____
11. Positive Attitude and Emotions	____	Air Pollution	____
12. Safe and Clean Environment	____	Soda or Store Juices	____
13. Meditation/Prayer Life	____	Snacks Between Meals	____
14. Purpose for Life	____	Processed or Junk Foods	____
15. Personal Responsibility for Health	____	Excessive TV (>10 Hrs./Wk.)	____
TOTAL MAXIMIZING FACTORS	_____	TOTAL MINIMIZING FACTORS	_____

COLUMN 1_____MINUS COLUMN 2_____= _____ (MY HQ SCORE)

SCORING	POINTS
Radiant Health	125 – 150
Optimum Health	100 – 125
Sub-optimum Health	60 – 100
Needs Improvement	< 60

103

Appendix B:
Personal Health Evaluation

The following statements provide a comprehensive picture of a person who has chosen to adopt health-giving habits in all areas of life. Read each statement and consider whether it is also true in your life.

Air

I breathe fresh clean air regularly

I avoid smoke-filled environments

I know how to breathe properly

I breathe through my diaphragm

I include deep breathing in my weekly exercise

I keep my environment free of chemicals and fumes

Water

I drink enough purified or distilled water

I avoid tap and chlorinated water

I avoid ice water

I shower or bathe regularly

I avoid harsh soaps, shampoos, and cleaning chemicals

I avoid carbonated beverages

I avoid caffeinated beverages

Nutrition

I eat fresh fruits and vegetables daily

I eat whole foods daily

I eat enough raw foods

I properly combine my foods

I eat simple, nourishing meals

I eat light dinners

I chew my food slowly and thoroughly

I allow 4 to 6 hours between meals

I eat only when I'm hungry

I eat in a peaceful and calm physical and healthy, emotional environment

I avoid liquids with meals I minimize my meat and dairy intake

I use nut milks and home-made rice milk instead of milk

I avoid over-the-counter supplements

I am careful to avoid refined and processed foods

I avoid refined sugar and sugar substitutes

I avoid foods with added chemicals and preservatives

I avoid tobacco, alcohol, caffeine, and drugs

Sunlight

I am exposed to sunshine 10-20 minutes daily, when available

I avoid overexposure to sunshine

Exercise and Activity

I get mild, comfortable exercise regularly

I use a variety of muscles when I exercise

I avoid over-exercise

I enjoy my exercise and activities

My work activity is free of anxiety and stress

My home life is calm, peaceful, and nurturing I exercise my body, mind, and spirit

Rest

I allow myself to rest when I need it

I allow myself enough sleep
(8 hours minimum)

I fast or juice to rest and rejuvenate my body and mind

Mental Outlook

I relax my mind from work and anxiety

I spend time alone each day
I love and accept myself

I enjoy my home and occupation I allow myself

playtime

I love and accept my neighbors and environment

I have a positive attitude about my health

I avoid anger, despair, sadness, guilt, and revenge

Spiritual Outlook

I have a spiritual understanding which provides peace and hope for my life

I emphasize love, hope, joy, peace, and forgiveness

I pray and meditate for guidance

Personal Responsibility
& Purpose in Life

I take personal responsibility for my health

I actively seek information about my health

I ask questions of my health practitioner and keep asking until I'm satisfied

I have a sense of purpose for my life and a feeling of well-being

I have personal goals that make my life worthwhile

I am living my life according to my deeper values

Appendix C:
Carbohydrate/Fat/Protein
Content of Selected Foods*

Food Item	Carbohydrate (% of calories)	Fat (% of calories)	Protein (% of calories)	Total Calories
Fruits				
Apple, raw 5 oz.	92	6	2	80
Apricot 4 oz.	90	7	3	51
Avocado 4 oz.	9	86	5	183
Banana 1 small - 4 oz.	90	5	5	105
Blueberries 1 cup - 4 oz.	92	7	1	64
Cantaloupe 1 cup cubes	83	7	10	56
Cherries, sweet 1 cup	81	12	7	104
Cherries, sour 1 cup	87	5	8	78
Cranberries 1 cup	95	2	3	46
Currants, bulk 1 cup	84	6	10	71

Food Item	Carbohydrate (% of calories)	Fat (% of calories)	Protein (% of calories)	Total Calories
Fruits				
Dates, 5 - approx. 1½ oz.	96	1	3	114
Fig, fresh *3 - approx. 3 oz.*	93	4	3	111
Fig, Dried *3 - approx. 2 oz.*	91	4	5	143
Grapefruit *1/2 – approx. 4 oz.*	89	3	8	39
Grapes, fresh *1 cup*	92	4	4	58
Honeydew *1 cup cubes*	92	3	5	60
Kiwi *1 - approx. 2½ oz.*	86	6	8	46
Lemon *1 - approx. 2 oz.*	76	9	15	16
Mango *1 - approx. 7 oz.*	93	4	3	134
Nectarine *1 - approx. 5 oz.*	84	9	7	67
Orange *1 - approx. 5 oz.*	91	2	7	76
Papaya *1 - approx. 6 oz.*	91	3	6	70
Peach *1 - approx. 4 oz.*	92	2	6	49
Pear *1 - approx. 6 oz.*	91	6	3	96
Persimmon *1- approx. 6 oz.*	95	2	3	118

Food Item	Carbohydrate (% of calories)	Fat (% of calories)	Protein (% of calories)	Total Calories
Fruits				
Pineapple, fresh *1 cup*	89	8	3	76
Plums *2 - approx. 4½ oz.*	85	10	5	73
Prunes *5 - approx. 1½ oz.*	94	2	4	100
Raisins *1/2 cup*	95	1	4	219
Strawberry *1 cup*	81	11	8	45
Watermelon *1 cup cubes*	80	12	8	51

Food Item	Carbohydrate (% of calories)	Fat (% of calories)	Protein (% of calories)	Total Calories
Vegetables				
Asparagus *1 cup boiled*	49	11	40	46
Bamboo shoots *1 cup slices*	45	19	36	25
Beets *4 oz. fresh*	85	2	13	50
Broccoli *fresh 4 oz.*	50	8	42	32
Cabbage, fresh *4 oz.*	73	7	20	27
Carrots, 1 raw *2 ½ oz.*	87	4	9	31
Cauliflower, raw *4 oz.*	60	6	34	27

Food Item	Carbohydrate (% of calories)	Fat (% of calories)	Protein (% of calories)	Total Calories
Vegetables				
Celery *1 cup diced, raw*	72	8	20	20
Chard *1 cup chopped*	59	4	37	36
Cucumber, raw *1/2 - 5 oz.*	75	9	16	20
Dandelion greens *4 oz.*	70	6	24	51
Eggplant *4 oz.*	80	4	16	29
Endive, raw *1 cup chopped*	59	11	30	8
Kale, fresh *4 oz.*	69	6	25	57
Lettuce *4 oz.*	56	13	31	20
Mushrooms *4 oz.*	50	16	34	28
M u s h r o o m s, Shitake, *4 oz.*	85	4	11	62
Okra *1 cup boiled*	74	3	23	52
Olives *4 oz.*	2	96	2	146
Onion, fresh *2/3 cup - 4 oz.*	79	7	14	39
Parsley *1/2 cup*	65	8	28	10
Potato *1 - approx. 7 oz.*	91	1	8	220

Food Item	Carbohydrate (% of calories)	Fat (% of calories)	Protein (% of calories)	Total Calories
Vegetables				
Pumpkin *1/2 cup, 4 oz.*	81	7	12	41
Spinach, fresh 4 oz.	38	10	52	25
Squash, butternut *4 oz.*	90	2	8	51
Squash, spaghetti, *1 cup*	84	8	8	45
Sweet potato *1 approx. 4 oz.*	93	1	6	117
Tomato *1 approx. 4 oz.*	69	14	17	26
Yam *1 approx. 4 oz.*	96	1	5	134

Food Item	Carbohydrate (% of calories)	Fat (% of calories)	Protein (% of calories)	Total Calories
Nuts and Seeds				
Almonds *1 oz.*	9	80	11	167
Brazil nuts *1 oz.*	2	91	8	186
Cashews *1 oz.*	18	73	9	163
Coconut, grated *1 oz.*	13	85	4	99
Macadamia *1 oz.*	3	95	2	199

Food Item	Carbohydrate (% of calories)	Fat (% of calories)	Protein (% of calories)	Total Calories
Nuts and Seeds				
Pecans 1 oz.	6	91	3	189
Pine nuts 1 oz.	4	89	7	146
Pumpkin seeds 1 oz. hulled	9	76	15	154
Sunflower seeds 1 oz.	10	76	14	162
Walnuts 1 oz.	7	87	6	182

Food Item	Carbohydrate (% of calories)	Fat (% of calories)	Protein (% of calories)	Total Calories
Grains				
Amaranth, raw seeds 1 cup	81	16	13	366
Barley 1 cup cooked	93	3	4	194
Brown rice 1 cup cooked	91	7	2	220
Corn 1 ear	85	11	4	83
Millet 1 oz. cooked	82	8	10	286
Oatmeal 3/4 cup cooked	81	15	4	109

Food Item	Carbohydrate (% of calories)	Fat (% of calories)	Protein (% of calories)	Total Calories
Legumes				
Adzuki *1 cup boiled*	79	1	20	294
Black beans *1 cup boiled*	72	4	24	228
Chickpeas *2 oz. raw*	67	11	22	204
Green peas *1 cup boiled*	76	2	22	134
Kidneys *1 cup boiled*	71	4	25	224
Lentils *1 cup boiled*	70	3	27	230
Lima *1 cup boiled*	76	3	21	212
Peanuts *1oz. dried*	8	78	16	161
Pink *1 cup boiled*	75	3	22	250
Pinto *1 cup boiled*	74	3	23	234
Soybeans *1 cup boiled*	20	47	35	298
Split pea *1 cup boiled*	72	3	25	232

Food Item	Carbohydrate (% of calories)	Fat (% of calories)	Protein (% of calories)	Total Calories
Flesh Foods**				
Bacon 4 oz.	0	77	23	653
Chicken 4 oz.	0	52	48	263
Duck 4 oz.	0	76	24	382
Hamburger 4 oz.	0	64	36	327
Ham, canned 4 oz.	0	62	38	215
Hot-dog 4 oz.	25	61	14	351
Leg of lamb 4 oz.	0	38	62	216
Lobster 4 oz.	2	14	84	101
Pork loin 4 oz.	0	54	46	292
Salmon, Coho 4 oz.	0	37	63	209
Sardines 4, 2 oz.	0	50	50	100
Sausage 4 oz.	0	82	18	449
Sirloin 4 oz.	0	35	67	221
Swordfish 4 oz.	0	30	70	176
Tuna 4 oz.	0	31	69	208

Food Item	Carbohydrate (% of calories)	Fat (% of calories)	Protein (% of calories)	Total Calories
Dairy and Eggs**				
Butter 4 oz.	0	100	0	813
Cheese 4 oz.	2	75	23	425
Cottage cheese 4 oz.	16	19	65	102
Cream cheese 4 oz.	2	90	8	396
Milk, Skim 8 oz.	57	4	39	80
Milk, Whole 8 oz.	29	52	19	146
Milk, 2% fat 8 oz.	39	35	26	114
Milk, 1% fat 8 oz.	46	23	31	96
Yogurt, plain, nonfat	58	0	42	56
Egg, raw 4 oz.	1	60	39	169

* Mostly from U.S. Dietary Guidelines, with similar recommendations from other sources (e.g., *Prevention* magazine's Nutrition Advisor, which uses other governmental sources). Carbohydrate, fat and protein sources have been rounded to the nearest digit. The purpose of this chart is to demonstrate relative content, not clinical accuracy.
** Not recommended. Included for comparison purposes only.

Appendix D:
Staples For Vegetarian Cooking And Eating

Fruits and Vegetables (preferably in season)

Apple	Lemons	Asparagus	Mustard greens
Apricot	Mango	Bamboo shoots	Okra
Avocado	Nectarines	Beets	Olives
Banana	Oranges	Broccoli	Onion
Blueberries	Papaya	Cabbage	Parsley
Cantaloupe	Peaches	Carrots	Pimento
Cherries	Pears	Cauliflower	Potato
Cranberries	Persimmons	Celery	Pumpkin
Currants	Pineapples	Collards	Spinach
Dates	Plums	Cucumber	Squash, Butternut
Figs	Prunes	Dandelion greens	Squash, Summer
Grapefruit	Raisins	Eggplant	Sweet Potato
Grapes	Strawberries	Endive	Tomatoes
Honeydew	Watermelon	Kale	Zucchini
Kiwi	Fruit juices	Lettuce	Vegetable juices

Nuts and Seeds, Raw and/or Soaked, as appropriate

Store nuts and seeds in refrigerator or freezer, or vacuum seal in jars.

Almonds	Hazelnuts	Sunflower seeds
Brazil nuts	Pecans	Walnuts
Cashews	Pine nuts	Almond butter, raw
Coconuts	Pumpkin seeds	Cashew butter, raw

Grains

Store grains in airtight jars or containers in the cupboard. To destroy insect eggs, place in the freezer for 48 hours before storing in a cupboard.

Amaranth	Corn	Whole grain spaghetti
Barley	Millet	Mixed grains
Buckwheat	Oats	Multi-grain/sprouted bread
Brown rice	Rye	Wheat berries

Flour

If you do not have a home flour mill, store flour in the refrigerator or freezer or in cool cupboard.

Barley flour	Oat flour	Semolina flour
Cornmeal	Rice flour	Whole wheat flour
Durum flour	Rye flour	Soy flour

Legumes

Black beans	Lentils	Pinto
Black eye peas	Lima	Soybeans
Garbanzos	Peanuts	Split pea
Kidneys	Pink or red beans	Mixed beans

Dried Fruits

Store dried fruits in an airtight container; Refrigerate or freeze. Cupboard storage is okay, if the dried fruits are sealed in jars. Naturally dried, organic fruit is best. Rinse sulfur from commercially dried fruits. Soak before using, if possible.

Apples	Coconut	Prunes
Apricots	Papaya	Raisins
Dates	Pineapples	Any others
Figs	Pears	

Cold/Hot Cereals

Amaranth flakes	Homemade granola	Mueseli ™
Oatmeal	7 Sprouted grains	Shredded wheat
Cream of Wheat™	Millet	Wheatena™
	Any other whole grain with no sugar or fruit added	

Vital Foods

Barley green	Brewers yeast	Wheat germ
Bee pollen	Chlorella	Wheatgrass
Blue-green algae	Spirulina	

Cooking Helpers

Arrowroot powder	Baking yeast	Homemade bread crumbs
Agar and Emes gelatin	Carob powder	Distilled water
Olive oil spray	Egg substitute	

Seasonings and Flavorings

Cayenne pepper	Garlic	Olive oil
Curry powder	Onion	Grape seed oil
Ginger	Cilantro	Homemade sauces

Herbs

Anise	Coriander	Onion flakes
Basil	Cumin	Oregano
Bay leaves	Dill weed	Paprika
Caraway seeds	Fennel seed	Parsley flakes
Cardamon	Italian seasoning	Thyme
Celery seed	Marjoram	Tumeric

Homemade Milk Substitutes

Almond milk	Rice milk	Grain milk
Cashew milk	Sesame milk	Seed milk

Herbal Caffeine Substitutes

Alfalfa tea	Ginseng root	Parsley tea
Chamomile tea	Ginger root	Peppermint tea
Chicory root	Goldenseal root	Kraft Postum™
Comfrey tea	Cafix	Red clover tea
Dandelion root	Lemongrass	Kaffree Roma

Appendix E:
Dietary Food Examples

The following are examples of live and whole food choices that are properly combined.

Breakfast

This is the most important meal of the day and should consist generally of fruits. Nuts and/or seeds can also be added. The amount eaten should be based on appetite and activity level. Take a glass of water to start the day (add lemon juice, if available or desired). Breakfast should be between 6 and 8 a.m.

1	Juice of 1/2 pineapple and/or 1 to 2 apples, and 1/2 lemon; any combination of almonds, pumpkin/sunflower seeds or celery filled with nut butter.	8	Fruit cocktail supreme: Any combination of oranges, strawberries, kiwi, apples, and grapes topped with 2 tablespoons of nut butter/cream or sesame seed topping.
2	3 to 5 oranges, small handful of almonds and/or pumpkin/sunflower seeds, celery.	9	Celery pieces stuffed with nut butter and raisins with optional nut and seed dried fruit trail mix.
3	Sweet fruit cocktail: 1 to 2 bananas, 3 figs, 3 dates, 2 prunes, raisins, celery.	10	Any combination of watermelon, cantaloupe, and honeydew melon.
4	Almond milk made by blending a handful of almonds in 8 oz. distilled water and dates or figs.	11	1 glass apple juice (with lemon, if desired), 1/2 pound grapes, 1/2 pound cherries.
5	Almond and berry juice: substitute strawberries, raspberries and /or blueberries for the orange above in breakfast number 2.	12	Steamed and sprouted vegetables with nuts and seeds or almond butter and a small salad.
6	Fruit cereal: Any combination of bananas, figs, apples, dates, or strawberries, blueberries, nuts, and apples with almond, sesame, or your favorite nut/seed milk.	13	Sprouted grain cereal with a rice , grain, or almond milk, 1 to 2 slices of whole grain toast (optional nut spread), 1 to 3 stalks of celery or cucumber slices.
7	Fruit cocktail: 1 peach, 3 apricots, 1 nectarine, 1 plum, 2 fresh figs, 1 banana with celery or cucumbers.	14	Oatmeal with rice or almond milk and wheat germ, with whole grain toast or whole grain toast/bagel with nut or avocado spread.

The digestion is strongest in the afternoon, and this is when the largest and most complex meal should be eaten. Other basic tips include the following:

- Lunch should generally be eaten at least 4 to 6 hours after breakfast.
- Only water, herbal tea (mint teas are especially good for aiding digestion), or juice should be taken between breakfast and lunch, at least 1 to 2 hours after breakfast or 30 minutes before lunch.
- No liquids should be taken with the meal.
- Vegetable juice can be taken 1/2 hour before lunch, e.g., tomato juice, carrot juice, cabbage juice, etc. One of my favorites is carrot, celery, and parsley juice (kale or chard, optional).

Lunch

The following meal combinations are suggested for lunch. Portions can be adjusted based on appetite and activity level.

1	Vegetable salad: Any combination of lettuce, tomato, cilantro, parsley, peppers, cucumbers, sprouts, radishes, onions, and garlic. Use virgin olive oil with or without lemon juice for dressing.	8	Vegetable or bean soup with a raw garden salad
2	Vegetable salad supreme: Add nuts, seeds, avocado and/or olives to Lunch No. 1	9	Black beans with onions and tomato sauce with a side of green vegetables and a small salad
3	Sandwich of mixed greens, tomato, avocado, and sprouts on sprouted grain toast, and a salad if still hungry	10	One slice of sprouted grain toast with eggplant spread, topped with avocado and tomato
4	Caesar salad without eggs. Vegetable minestrone soup	11	Brown rice with lightly steamed vegetables and a garden salad
5	Baked potato, small garden salad, and green vegetables; e.g., broccoli, cauliflower, peas	12	Chinese deluxe vegetables, steamed vegetarian pot stickers and a small salad
6	Brown rice, raw corn on the cob or mixed greens and garden salad	13	Whole grain pasta with whole tomato sauce, peppers, and onions, with a small salad
7	Garden salad with steamed vegetables: any combination of broccoli, carrots, mushrooms, onions, peppers, zucchini, and squash	14	Brown rice tostada with assorted vegetables, guacamole dip with fresh, organic, unsalted corn chips, and a small garden salad

Only water, herbal teas, or juice, sipped slowly, should be taken between lunch and dinner, at least 2 hours after the meal.

Dinner

Dinner should be the lightest meal of the day, if eaten at all. Ideally, it should be eaten by 6:00 PM at least 3 hours before going to bed (fruit, 1 to 2 hours) to ensure that the stomach is empty. Any downsized portions of the breakfast or lunch examples can be selected. The following are some examples of recommended simple, nutritious dinner choices:

1	Salad with steamed vegetables	6	Sub-acid fruit salad: apples, peaches, pears, plums, cherries, and/or grapes
2	Salad with brown rice or potatoes	7	Sweet fruit salad: bananas, figs, dates, prunes
3	Garden salad	8	Salad with sprouted whole-grain toast
4	Acid fruit salad: Oranges, strawberries, kiwi, with celery	9	Fruit juice Small fruit cocktail
5	Melon salad	10	Vegetable juice or broth with small garden salad and zwieback or sprouted grain toast

Herbal tea, e.g., chamomile, valerian, hops, ginger, comfrey, red clover, pau d'arco, can be taken before bed.

The optimum diet for most people is a highly complex carbohydrate, low fat, and low protein diet with sufficient calories. This provides all the vitamins, minerals, fats, and proteins required for optimum health. The best foods are raw, live foods, but for practical purposes, a reasonable goal of 75 percent raw and 25 percent cooked may offer the best results (except in the case of cancer, where a 100 percent raw food diet may be best). Any dietary transition should take place over a period of time, starting with one raw, live food meal per day and working up to the 75/25 percent goal. Working with a qualified health professional is an excellent way to assist you in taking your current diet and adapting it to your desired goals based on your current state of health, activity level, and lifestyle characteristics.

Creative, whole-food sauces, dressings, and combinations can be added to the above examples for variety and taste. In general, however, the diet should be simple, nutritious, and completely satisfying.

Appendix F:
References and Suggested Readings

Author	Title(s)
Becker, Robert O., M.D.	*The Body Electric*
Boutenko, Victoria	*12 Steps to Raw Foods*
Chamberlin, Katy	*Something Better – God's Original Design*
Clark, Hulda Regehe, Ph.D., N.D.	*A Cure for All Cancers A Cure for All Diseases*
Cousins, Norman	*Anatomy of an Illness*
Diamond, Harvey and Marilyn	*Fit For Life Fit For Life II*
Duke, James A., Ph.D.	*Herbs of the Bible The Green Pharmacy*
Ferrell, Vance	*Natural Remedies Encyclopedia*
Foster, Vernon W, M.D.	*New Start!*
Fuhrman, Joel, M.D.	*Fasting and Eating for Health*
Haas, Elson M., M.D.	*A Diet for All Seasons* *Staying Healthy with Nutrition The Detox Diet*
Huxley, Aldous	*The Art of Seeing*
Jensen, Bernard, D.C.	*Foods that Heal Chemistry of Man*
Klaper, Michael, M.D.	*A Diet for All Reasons*
Kloss, Jethro Loomis, Howard F. D.C., F.I.A.C.A.	*Back to Eden* *Enzymes: The Key to Health Vol. 1*
Malkmus, Dr. George A.	*God's Way to Ultimate Health*
McDougall, John A., M.D.	*A Challenging Second Opinion The McDougal Program*
Mendelsohn, Robert S., M.D.	*Confessions of a Medical Heretic*
Miller, Neil Z.	*Vaccines: Are they Really Safe and Effective?*
Morter, Jr., Dr. M. Ted	*Fell's Know-It-All Guide to Health & Wellness*
Nedley, Neil, M.D.	*Proof Positive*
Nilson, Paul	*Raw Knowledge Raw Knowledge II The Raw Life*

Author	Title(s)
Rector-Page, N.D., Ph.D.	*Healthy Healing*
Robbins, John	*Diet For A New America*
Schneider, Meir, Ph.D.	*Self-Healing: My Life and Vision* *The Handbook for Self-Healing*
Shelton, Herbert M.	*Fasting Can Save Your Life* *Food Combining Made Easy*
Shook, Edward, D.C.	*Advanced Treatise in Herbology*
Shorter, Gwen & Rick	*Sister Shorter's Health Manual*
Thrash, Agatha, M.D.	*Home Remedies and Hydrotherapy* *Nutrition For Vegetarians*
Turley, Susan, M.A.,B.S.N., RN, RHIT, CMT	*Medical Language*
Weil, Andrew, M.D.	*Health and Healing* *Natural Health, Natural Medicine* *Spontaneous Healing*
White, Ellen G.	*Counsels on Diet and Foods* *Counsels on Health* *Ministry of Healing*

Other Reference Materials

Title	Publisher
Alternative Medicine	The Burton Goldberg Group
CELEBRATIONS	General Conference of Seventh-day Adventists
Definitive Guide to CANCER	W. John Diamond, M.D., W. Lee Cowden, M.D.
Encyclopedia of Medicine	American Medical Association
Physicians' Desk Reference	Medical Economics Data
The PDR Pocket Guide	Medical Economics Company
The Holy Bible	

Feedback and Personal Notes

Personal Notes

Health Challenges, Concerns or Questions	Health Goals and Objectives	Short and Lon-term Plans

To learn more about the principles outlined in this book, or to receive a Certificate or Degree, you may enroll in our school, The International Institute of Original Medicine.

The International Institute of Original Medicine (IIOM) is a Christian distance-learning educational institute. Our intent is to provide health education and offerings that are in harmony with the Creator's natural laws of health. We believe that our offerings provide our Christian and non-Christian students, with a powerful set of time-honored principles and techniques for developing the whole person – body, mind and spirit. We are a dynamic organization, building an ever-growing network of health professionals and affiliations to ensure the highest quality education to meet the needs of our valued students.

IIOM provides a full spectrum of offerings designed to empower personal self-improvement and professional aspirations. Our courses give you a deeper appreciation of how we are fearfully and wonderfully made in the image and likeness of God. We are confident that you will find our program to be one of the most diversified natural healing programs available in the 21st century.

Certificate programs   Nutrition Counselor, Herbalist, and Medical Missionary

Degree Programs   Bachelor's, Master's, Doctorate

Contact Information
www.iiomonline.com ~ (410) 884-9319

For additional information, questions or an appointment to develop a *personalized health strategy* based on the principles outlined in this book, contact us at:

International Institute of Original Medicine
P. O. Box 311
Smithfield, VA 23431
(410) 884-9319 (phone)
(757)3573388 (fax)
Web site:www.iiomonline.com
E-mail: info@iiomonline.com

"Whether you eat or drink or whatever you do, do all for the glory of God."
– 1Corinthians 10:31

Through this book, which outlines my philosophy to attain optimum health through the harmonious integration of body, mind, and spirit, may you be blessed in starting or accelerating your journey toward an empowered and healthy life.

– Dr. Jim Sharps

www.ingramcontent.com/pod-product-compliance
Lightning Source LLC
Chambersburg PA
CBHW041427270326
41932CB00030B/3486